Blessing Love

A Widow's Story

Judy Brutz

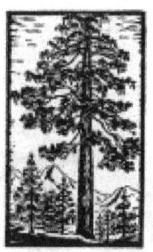

Pine River Press
Pocatello, Idaho

Author's photo by artist George Wise
Book Design by Judy Brutz
Book Cover by Judy Brutz

ISBN-13: 978-1492768555
ISBN-10: 1492768553

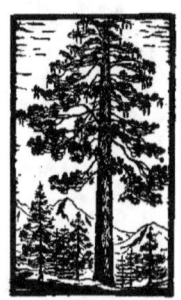

Pine River Press
Pocatello, Idaho

Other Books by Judy Brutz

Abuse Survivors: Self-Guided Retreat, a Memoir of Healing
ISBN - 13: 9780984851003
ISBN - 10: 0984851003

Crying Out to God in the Manner of the Lord's Prayer
ISBN -13: 9780984851027
ISBN -10: 0978098451027

Table of Contents

In Memory

David Brutz
1937 – 2011

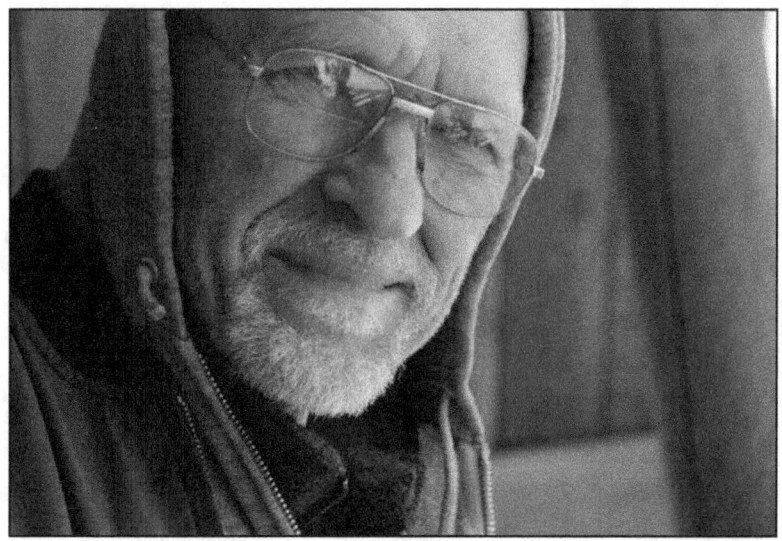

Photo by Judy Brutz

Preface

"None of us know where our spiritual journey will take us, or which twists and turns will occur. I do know that my journey deepens my faith and closeness to God and that my living Love is my lifelong path."

From the author of *Blessing Love, a Widow's Story*, this intimate memoir of loss, grief, self-discovery, and growth will resonate deeply with every woman who has ever mourned the death of a husband and questioned her own purpose.

Judy Brutz shares her last sixteen months of life with her husband while he was dying from brain cancer and at the same time she was being treated for Hepatitis C. Their fifty year marriage had the usual ups and downs of marital problems, and yet, underneath they continued to share a deep and abiding love and a spiritual bond which saw them through difficulties and blossomed into full maturity in their last months side-by-side.

Theirs is the story of hope, joy and the healing of a relationship. After David's passing the blessing of their love continues as Judy faces questions of "Who am I?" and asks, "David, help me."

Judy Brutz PhD inspires deepening spirituality through stories, prayers, and memoir. She draws from her experience and gifts as Spiritual Director, Hospice Chaplain, Marriage and Family Therapist, and mentor for Education of Ministry (EfM).

Author of:
Abuse Survivors: Self-guided Retreat, a Memoir of Healing
Crying out to god, In the Manner of the Lord's Prayer

Blessing Love, A Widow's Story

It's a story of our love: we were married for fifty years and we shared life's struggles, pains and joys, and we shared his diminishment too, then he died.

A few months after he was gone and the worst of settling affairs was over, I figured I could return to my writing. I walked around my new apartment and it was our library that drew me in – David's bird books, his binoculars, and his geology texts and maps were next to my books on writing, spirituality, Quakerism and knitting. My hands reached out for *"Kaufman's Field Guide."* I paged through and came to the entry on Sage-Grouse. When I was well enough we had gone on a field trip with the bird club to view the displaying male Sage-Grouse busy courting the females who appeared to care less. I held the book close. I felt so alone and at such a loss. I asked David out loud, *"Who am I? What am I supposed to do? David, help me."* I had always been able to count on David to stand by me. Further, I was the risk-taker and he was my anchor. Grief calls you out and challenges you to find vitality.

PART I - TWO NATIONAL CRISES
Love comforts

Two National Crises

April 30, 2013 Tuesday – Pocatello, Idaho

Two weeks have passed since the Boston Marathon bombing. That day I was glued to CNN's coverage. The images kept playing over: the man who fell down and the woman just ahead of him, turning her head to look and continuing to run; the police, the first responders, the blood, the two blasts, the smoke, the photos of the two suspected brothers from where? Who were they and why? Could this all be real?

I don't know how long I stared at the TV screen. I was numb and frightened. On that day I desperately needed my husband, but he was gone. David died one and a half years ago.

Oh my dear love I long for your arms.

I feel closely tied to Boston. WE WERE MARRIED IN BOSTON. Our apartment on Beacon Hill was close to the finish line of The Marathon. Our first baby was born in Boston. The Boston Marathon Crisis for me ignited a memory of an earlier national crisis.

The Cuban Missile Crisis

I was four and a half months pregnant at the time of this national crisis. I was terrified as the news came over the news wires. My breathing was shallow. I felt like crying hysterically but I suppressed all my tears.

"What are we going to do? Where can we go to be safe?" I questioned. I believed we were headed into World War III which was going to be fought on our continent not in Europe. No place would be safe since the Cuban-Soviet missiles could reach us in Boston, a sure-fire target. Our job was to keep our unborn baby safe.

David was not one to show panic. He held me, his hand on my pregnant belly. I told him my fears. He listened lovingly. We became quiet. Our stillness was prayer.

Love comforts.

PART II – HEALING

Healing is a mystery - we may ask why is one person healed and not another? We may wonder at the end of someone's life why there hasn't been a cure of the disease, and yet there has been healing of relationships and in the person's closeness to the Holy One.

1

People, who haven't seen me for a while, can't believe their eyes. Folks generally exclaim, "You're walking! What happened? You were in an electric scooter and were on oxygen. . ."

I was so sick with what had been diagnosed as Parkinson's, I almost died. We were beginning to talk to hospice. I had a hospital bed and was on oxygen twenty-four hours a day. One Saturday I realized that I no longer had quality of life. I couldn't face lying there helplessly not being able to enjoy life any longer and not knowing how long the decline would be. I decided to stop taking my meds. I didn't tell my family. They would have had a fit, particularly my husband.

To my surprise, every day I improved.

On the sixth day, I walked into my neurologist's office without assistance and without oxygen. She took one look at me, "Obviously you do not have Parkinson's."

Parkinson's is very difficult to diagnose. Several neurologists had seen me and they were united in saying that I didn't have the typical profile. Yes, I had the tremor. Yes, I was hunched over and shuffled my feet, and my balance was off. Further when I was given the meds, my symptoms lessoned. It turned out that I was misdiagnosed. We didn't find out what the culprit was until May of 2010.

That May was very difficult. **Within the same month we received two diagnoses that would radically change our lives.**

On May 1st, I was diagnosed as having Hepatitis C. The information was too much to take in. How could I have Hepatitis C? Would I die from it? What was going to happen next?

My internist, Dr. Gilbert, made the diagnosis. My blood work had shown that there was something going on with my liver and the test for Hep C was positive.

Later I learned that the virus strain was genotype 1b with a viral load of 4,500,000 IU/ml. This type is resistant to treatment and the treatment is likely to include a protocol of Interferon injections. The side effects could include muscle pain, chills, fever, severe headaches, nausea, vomiting, loss of appetite and loss of hair and extreme fatigue. I had hopes that acupuncture and Chinese herbal medicine would reduce the side effects.

Resistant to treatment means that the virus can cause serious liver disease such as cirrhosis of the liver and liver cancer. Sometimes part of the liver can be removed if the disease is in one area. Sometimes liver transplants are recommended. What was going to happen? Was I rid of one diagnosis whose toxic meds just about killed me to instead have liver disease which was far more life threatening?

My immediate worries were how I was to cope. How was I to continue writing since I was gearing up to have my first book published? How was I going to be able to lead my week-long workshop in July at the annual Gathering of Friends General Conference to take place in Ohio?

Dr. Gilbert scheduled an appointment with a gastroenterologist who would be able to provide treatment. I saw the physician assistant who informed me that I was too old to take treatment and I believed him. I was 69 years old.

David was absolutely insistent that I should be treated. We went together to see Dr. Gilbert.

Dr. Gilbert quietly asked, "Aren't they even going to do a biopsy?"

His question tipped me off that he strongly disagreed with the opinion that I was too old for treatment. Dr. Gilbert obtained an appointment for the following week with the Liver Clinic at the University of Utah Medical Center. David drove us down to the appointment, about a three hour drive, one-way. David seemed calm and like the rest of our life together, was there for me.

It was the last week in May by the time I saw Dr. Kerin Stevens in the Liver Clinic for consultation. I was ready to be educated and Kerin told me that I probably received the virus in 1985 when I had surgery. Blood was not yet being screened and furthermore it was the era when if you bled during an operation, blood transfusions were freely given. Treatment would involve self-injections of Interferon and an oral anti-virus medication. She let me know that the treatment would make me very sick with lowered immune system, skin breakdown, anemia and nausea. She told me about the Interferon fog which affects one's ability to think. In addition, I was going to feel weak and that I was probably going to spend half the week laying low.

I asked Kerin, she preferred being called by her first name, to follow me as her patient. She agreed and faxed the prescription for Interferon to our home-town pharmacy. My first self-injection was the beginning of June.

David, my dear heart, wanted us to move to Salt Lake so that I would be close to the University Hospitals and he initiated our looking for housing there but the air quality was so ghastly that we quickly gave up that idea. Instead we made the rounds of assisted living places in Pocatello just in case I might need to receive care. We made the rounds; places differed greatly. Some were old, dark, and none of the residents were out of their rooms. In others, residents were involved in activities and talking together. One was next to a shopping mall while another was on the mountain side and had a spectacular vista. Little did we know what was about to happen.

We saw Kerin a few days before Memorial Day Weekend. Little did we know what was coming next.

At the end of May, we learned that David had a brain tumor.

During the month of May, David was beginning to show some kind of neurological symptoms relating to his remembering words. This was a sudden change. Our daughter, Paula, who is a PA took notice and spoke to David's primary doctor. Immediately David had an MRI. This occurred on Saturday morning of Memorial Day Weekend. David and I were called to the doctor's office in the early afternoon. We didn't even make it into his office. He met us just inside the building's entrance. The building was closed and no one was around. We were invited to sit on the ledge of the building's tall window.

David's physician, standing in front of us, looked straight into my husband's eyes. "The MRI shows that you have some kind of tumor in your language area. You need to be seen by a surgeon right away. Would you like me to make you an appointment?"

We agreed that we wanted David to be seen by a surgeon in Salt Lake. David's doctor, bless him, made an appointment for the following Thursday with Dr. Fultz, the director of the department.

The whole family went into emergency mode. Our daughter obtained a copy of the MRI and she drove us to the appointment for the consultation with the surgeon. I was so thankful she was with us. With her expertise as a P.A. she had an in-depth discussion with the surgeon while they looked at the MRI. They discussed a diagnosis of Glioblastoma Multiforme, whatever that was.

David and I sat there, taking it all in the best we could. Frankly, I believe we were both in a state of shock. How could this be? What does it mean? Now what? In the coming days, I wasn't aware of much. David and I cuddled quietly, but the rest was a blur.

The family gathered, our daughter living locally and our son Philip from Ohio. I'm not sure how we traveled to Salt Lake.

Did we go in Paula's van with Philip driving or did Philip rent a vehicle? We stayed in the Guest House on campus in adjoining rooms, sister and brother in one room and David and I in the other. I don't remember taking sustenance only that we gently held each other through the night.

No, now I remember. Our oldest Granddaughter, Heather, met her dad Philip somewhere, though I don't recall whether they flew together or what. Heather would have come from the Washington D.C. area while Philip flew from Cleveland, Ohio. Philip rented a vehicle and the four of us drove to Salt Lake. Paula drove separately, but the picture is still very foggy. Did Paula and Heather sleep in one bed and Philip in the other? That makes sense, that's probably how it was.

Morning came, we arrived in the surgical waiting room, and many families were there with the one who was to have surgery. When David's name was called, it was Philip who went with his dad to the prep area. I felt comforted that Philip was the one to go with David. I was already on Interferon and was foggy and fatigued.

Then the waiting began. How long? I don't know. We were called to the recovery room at some point.

David's bed was rolled up to keep him in a semi-sitting position. His head was bandaged in gauze. His face was swollen and he was either asleep or had not yet regained consciousness. There was blood on the bandage and some kind of drain. He had IVs going. I could hardly breathe. Would he live? All that mattered was that I was near him. Just about everything remained a blur. I do know that we drove David back to Pocatello within a matter of days. Before going home, however, he needed to be at Quinn Meadows Rehabilitation and Care facility in Pocatello for recovery, where the Physical Therapists worked with him twice a day and he had round-the-clock care.

In the afternoons I would come and visit and lie with him in his narrow bed. It reminded me of our early marriage when we shared a twin bed. We either spooned or he would lie on his back with his knees bent and I would lie on my side, place my head on his shoulder, arm across his chest and my knees under his legs. Those were fond times.

In the meantime, many family hands, including mine, were knitting white cotton caps to keep David's head warm and to cover the incision. David was comforted.

2

There was a swirl of appointments at the Cancer Center in Pocatello and I drove him to all of them. David was to have targeted radiation followed by chemotherapy.

Patients who have radiation to the head have a special mask made. A mold is made of the face, and then a hard mesh mask is constructed. When the patient lies down on the platform, the mask is screwed in place so there won't be the slightest movement.

I searched the internet for information on Glioblastoma Multiforme. When it is diagnosed, it is already a stage four cancer. There is no cure, treatable yes, survivable no. It is an aggressive form of cancer. The life expectancy is short. We were given a prognosis of three to six months. Connectors between cells throughout the brain, called Glias, are not able to be excised and spread the cancer from the original tumor.

Research indicates that patients with brain cancer affecting their language area may be helped with speech therapy. I obtained an appointment for him. The speech therapy was helpful for a while. Also, I located a place in the south which was doing experimental treatment for Glioblastoma. Of course, David was interested, but his cancer had progressed too far.

David was a strong believer in "you do everything possible to stay alive." While I didn't share this conviction, I was going to support him in any way I could.

In the meantime, my treatment for Hep C was taking its toll. Weekly, I injected myself with Interferon and also took an antiviral medication orally. Interferon has serious side effects such as breakdown of skin, anemia and "interferon fog." For several days after the injection, I wouldn't be able to think straight and I was very weak. I managed taking David to his appointments, but the rest of the day I was wiped out.

3

The family cared deeply about their Father and Grandfather. They were concerned he might not receive quality care-giving from me. They were united in counseling me not to take treatment for Hep C so that I would be fully available to David. The message was that I could live a long time with a diseased liver, even if it became cirrhotic. David stood firm that I was to be treated, though I don't know if he informed the family of his views. It may be that I didn't disclose to him what was being said to me.

Before we moved to Pocatello from Des Moines Iowa, our daughter found us an apartment. I was declining with what was thought to be Parkinson's and we wanted to be close to Paula. We were all thrilled because it meant that our granddaughters, Megan and Julia, could come to us after school. David, who loved volunteering, went to the school to listen to children read to him one-on-one.

We continued living in our two bedroom apartment on S. Arthur Street for almost a year after the surgery. It was next to the Greenway which ran atop of an embankment just above Portneuf River. The Greenway path is used by walkers, runners, and bicyclists. Following that path we could walk to our granddaughters' school, the Pocatello Charter School.

Later in June of 2010 when David was in assisted living I moved to Cardona Senior Apartments, which offers independent housing for seniors.

4

How to care for the two of us was a real issue. Our daughter hired Linda to clean our apartment every other week. Linda did cleaning jobs while her kids were in school. She did the basics, dusting, vacuuming, and cleaning the kitchen floor, the counter tops and sink, along with the bathroom. Regardless, the clutter kept growing. It was not her job. My thinking was so compromised and my energies were so low there was no way that I could do the organization.

David insisted on driving, but it soon became clear that he wasn't safe.

He listened to his oncologist say, "You can't drive anymore because it is not safe."

"What if I drive slower?"
(Not, that he wasn't already driving slowly!)

"No. You don't want to be responsible for an accident and Judy is quite capable of driving."

The problem was when I was driving, David became highly anxious. *"You've got to drive more in the middle because someone might open their car door or a child might run out between cars!"*

To which I responded, "David, it isn't safe to drive over the center line."

I don't know how many go-a-rounds we had. But it was similar to a pattern that developed in the previous ten years when we lived in Des Moines. We were in our first owned home, purchased in our middle years.

David came in the side door saw me loading the dishwasher, *"No, that's not the way to order them."*

"David! Don't tell me how to do things. You have your way and I have mine. Neither is right or wrong."

He didn't like my response and he went back outside to become busy with something.

In those days our relationship became very strained. We gave each other the silent treatment. I had an opportunity to take part-time employment as a chaplain with Hospice of North Iowa. I would drive up to Mason City and stay overnight between two days of work. This gave us some distance from each other, some breathing space. We each looked forward to being together again and we re-ignited our love life.

Those two years as a chaplain were precious. Being with terminally ill people was such a gift. It amazed me how people would accept me into their homes or room, I a perfect stranger, and reveal their most intimate thoughts, feelings and memories. Little did I know that my experience would help me be with David during his last few months.

As both David and I were declining, it was clear to me that we needed home health care and I visited the Agency on Aging. With their references I found an agency that came in and did an assessment. Since I wasn't housebound we couldn't receive services for someone to cook or go shopping. They did stretch the rules and allowed LPNs to do things like check our vitals and cut our toenails. When this ended I'm not sure. From that ending until the family conference that would take place is just a blur.

Leading up to the conference, both David and I were really sick. I can't remember when David had a second brain surgery. It helped his ability to process and to communicate though it didn't last too long.

David was becoming more agitated. Whenever I would say something to him, his likely response was, *"I'm not going to argue."* He was angry. I obviously was not one to reason with him and I didn't know how to redirect him. We became quite distant from one another.

David's oncologist observed the dynamics between us since David would turn on me if I said anything at all during his appointments. Perhaps his observations led the Cancer Center's social worker to call a family conference.

5

It seems to me the conference was in September or October of 2010. Sitting around the table was the social worker at one end of a small rectangular table. To his left was Paula and next the oncologist. Facing the oncologist on our side of the table was Philip, then David and then me.

The social worker recommended that David go into assisted living since he needed more care than could be provided at home. Our son and daughter were vehemently opposed. David and I were silent.

The oncologist turned to Paula, "Are you going to hang your mother out on the line to dry?"

As the discussion continued, I turned more inward. I felt helpless and couldn't fathom why our son and daughter were taking the position they were.

Finally I turned to David and took his hand. We looked into each others' eyes, "David, what I really want is for you to go into assisted living. Please do it for me."

He responded, *"Of course."*

There we were - we stood together. Together we made the decision. We were one. It was our place to make such a choice.

***

When we left the conference and were outside in fresh air, Philip clarified that they were trying to preserve my financial resources. I explained to Philip and Paula that we had long-term healthcare insurance. They didn't know this because David and I had not communicated with them at the time we took out the insurance some ten years earlier. One of my regrets is that as parents we failed to disclose important information once our kids were on their own.

6

It was near the end of December that Paula approached me. She suggested, "You know, when people are terminally ill, they are comforted by the rituals of their childhoods. Bring Dad and come to Evening Mass at St. John's. Join us and the girls."

David was still home and we were lying together, "David, Paula is inviting us to come to Mass with her and the girls at St. John's on Sunday nights. Would you like to go?"

Oh my, did he become vocal. He was angry and surprisingly his English was fluent and grammatically correct. He ranted about the Catholic Church and how they didn't accept gays and lesbians, how they were opposed to birth control and worst of all how they were undoing Vatican II.

He had tears rolling down his cheeks, *"Pope John* (the XXIII) *was a humanitarian, and he accepted everyone. And now the church is trying to undo all the advances of Vatican II."*

I held him close and we were quiet for a while, "You know David, there is the Episcopal Church. They accept everyone. Everyone is welcomed to receive communion and they ordain women. Would you like to go there with me?"

"Yes." We cuddled and comforted each other.

David moved into assisted living and I reminded him that I would come on Sunday morning to take him to Trinity Episcopal Church. The first Sunday we went was on January 6th, the day of Epiphany. We found two seats at the end of a pew with David sitting on the end.

The music was so beautiful, the choir, many of whom were on the musical faculty at Idaho State University, filled the sanctuary with glorious sound, harmony reverberating through the sanctuary.

David had trouble reading, but by tracing my finger under the words, he was able to sing. Most of his adult life he sang in choruses and choirs, the last place being in the Community Choir of Drake University in Des Moines, Iowa. He never had voice lessons, he learned from his choir work. He had a beautiful tenor voice. I loved to hear him sing.

Every December wherever we lived, we would participate in the community Handel's Messiah. This was how we celebrated our anniversary. Our anniversary was on December 9th. David sang in the tenor section and I in the soprano.

At Trinity that Epiphany morning, David thrilled with the music and being able to sing. When it was time for communion, David stepped out into the aisle for the communicants to pass through.

"David, everyone can receive communion here. Would you like to go with me to receive?"

I took his arm and we went to the communion rail together. David knelt down and he knew to hold his hands to receive the bread and to drink from the cup. I stood beside him because I wasn't able to kneel.

The members of the church embraced us. We were welcomed and cared for from the very beginning.

I continued taking him for a few weeks, but he was declining rapidly. He forgot how to receive communion and was helped by me or the server. The last time he was able to go, he remembered what to do from his childhood. You receive the host on your tongue but you do not drink from the cup.

After that particular Sunday, he no longer was able to go because he had become socially inappropriate. If he needed to relieve himself, he was likely to mistake a wastebasket as a toilet that he could pee in.

PART III – TRANSITION

Transitions are markers between what has been and what will be. Transitions are hard, there is much confusion about identity, goals and even whether to live or not.

7 August 26, 2011 Friday

I haven't written for some time. I feel suspended, not really present in what I'm doing because my thoughts go to David. Yet for my own health I can't be with him around the clock.

Well, I was already ill. Was I going to survive Hep C? The Hospice social worker reminds me that I must take care of myself and that the surviving spouse is will become ill six to nine months after a spouse's passing

Two days earlier this week David asked Paula to stay overnight. We, Paula and I, decide for her not to.

Two days ago David is trying to tell me something. He is weak and his voice is hard to hear.

"I'm sorry..." and he doesn't continue. I'm trying to figure out what he's sorry about.

"Are you sorry about something in our marriage?"

"No" he replies.

"Are you leaving? I ask.

"No." he says firmly, *"just the opposite."*

I realize he is taking the meaning of my question to be about leaving the marriage.

He makes several attempts at saying he is sorry. Then, *"I'm sorry the disease grows."*

"Yes, David, your disease grows."

Minutes later he manages to communicate, *"I'll meet you in Heaven."*

"Yes David, I will meet you in Heaven. I love you David."

Tears are trickling from my eyes as we lay side-by-side holding hands. He is saying goodbye.

David is no longer able to feed himself and I feed him usually once a day. Last week I was irritated at the aides who claimed David liked the attention of my feeding him. In his wheelchair he sat with his back to them while they sat at the table where they feed or prompt people to eat. He is seated at the table where people could feed themselves and the aides were not observing that he needed help and supervision. He was helpless.

I told the Hospice nurse about the problem and she arranged for him to sit at the table where the aides sit. Now they see and understand.

They are understaffed for the number of residents who need assistance. So many of the people in this locked ward need more assistance than they are receiving and the director does not add any additional staff.

I'm with David four or five hours per day and I am drained.

This morning I was present when the Hospice nurse visited. His vital signs are stable. We discuss the dosage of Atavan he is receiving. I'm concerned because it seems to me that the medicine is causing him to be confused. She decides to keep him on the full dose at night because he sleeps better and then have a half dose in the morning. She is ordering the pharmacy to bubble wrap the half dose.

The Hospice nurse gently tells me, "David's confusion is due to the disease progression. He's not overdosed with Atavan."

This is a relief to hear in some ways since because I see that he's declining. I wonder will he still be with us when Philip visits on Labor Day Weekend. There is no way of predicting. We are going to take one day at a time, sometimes by one block of time to the next.

There is the issue of the deep thrombosis in the upper part of his left leg. The leg kept swelling until the aides placed his legs on Paula's rolled up down quilt either while he is sitting in his recliner or when he is laying in bed. His nurse measures his legs and is pleased the swelling has gone down on his lower leg.

47

While I'm feeding David at lunch today, he pulls his plate towards himself and begins to raise it. *"David, you need to leave the plate on the table."*

At one point, he lifts the table cloth and puts it in his mouth, and so it goes. My heart aches for him.

After lunch while we are lying in bed together holding hands, *"Judy I want you to take me hand-in-hand and tell me the truth of what is happening."* I'm surprised by how lucid he is.

"David, I will. We will be holding hands until you go to Heaven."

"Amen," he answers in a strong voice.

He is sleeping now. He is coughing quite a bit and I hear congestion. *"Dear love, be comfortable,"* a prayer as well as a statement to him.

"Thank you, Judy."

8 August 27, 2011 Saturday

When I asked David if he wanted me to pray with him, he said yes. David was sitting in his recliner. I had brought him his rosary and placed it in his hand. We were quiet together. He had me take it home. He wanted to make sure that I had it.

I noticed that the aides had not rolled up the down quilt and placed it under his feet. I rolled it up and asked the aides to help lift his legs.

Each time an aide comes on duty after a break of a week or more, she has to be educated. The communication doesn't carry over. They are too busy and they do well to keep track of what they are doing at the moment.

David asks me to spend the night. I ask if it is all right for me to sleep in the recliner, and he agrees. I go home and return around 9 pm. He is sleeping. I say hello and he recognizes my voice.

At the start of the night, I'm in the recliner. It was so uncomfortable that I went into his bed. To my surprise, we were both comfortable. He is no longer rolling and moving around like he did at the beginning of the year.

A conversation of note came earlier in the day. I remind David that Philip will be here next weekend and it will be Philip's birthday.

"David, is there something you would like to give Philip for his birthday?"

No response.

"Is there something you would like me to give?"

No response.

"David, you leave your legacy. Do you know what 'legacy' means?"

"Say the word again."

"Legacy means what you leave your family after you are gone. Your legacy to Philip is your values. You showed Philip how to be a good father and husband. You showed him how to be a good citizen and how to be a good neighbor. You give him the gift of who you are."

"Thank you Judy."

"And you leave the same gift to Paula."

We are quiet for a while.

"David, you have helped me to be a better person. You accept me as I am. Your love has helped me to become more like you, to be more patient and to be moderate in what I do. Thank you."

"You're welcome."

Before I leave he asks me to take the rosary home. He didn't want anything to happen to it and I think he wanted me to have it.

9 August 29, 2011 Monday

I'm finding it hard to eat. This morning, I drank Ensure and ate a piece of whole wheat toast, which has 5 grams of fiber in it.

The stress is taking its toll with eating problems and cramping that goes from my stomach to my throat. When the cramping occurs it is accompanied by an intense pain behind the breast bone. When I was in the rehab and care center, my doctor prescribed a medication for gastro reflux. I still have some bubble wrapped and started taking one a day. I do find relief, but it wears off by nighttime.

When I went to the med tray this morning, I had difficulty figuring out which of the morning pills I needed to take before eating. It should be levothyroxine and omeprazole. In my lack of focus, I think instead that I took buspar and pradaxa.

I crawled in bed and slept and decided not to answer the phone and thankfully no one called. However, I did get up to pay my rent and then go to the care facility to pay that bill.

When I checked in with David, they had him at the table to eat lunch.

David cannot have paper napkins anymore because he tears strips off and puts them in his mouth to eat. I fed him and tears were rolling down both his cheeks. I asked him what his tears were about, but he made no reply. As I think about it, I was being insensitive to ask such a question.

10   August 30, 2011 Tuesday

After doing Physical Therapy this morning, I arrived at 10 am at the care facility. David was in bed, his legs flat. He had not been showered, and the Hospice CNA left a note that David 'still NEEDS body wash and shampoo.' This info was news to me. I circled the note and wrote in the margin Okay and initialed it.

Upon lifting the covers to look at David's legs, I noticed a few things. Both ankles were swollen, the left much more. The bottoms of his feet were dry, cracked and peeling.

He enjoys my massaging his feet with lotion, and then continuing to hydrate his lower legs and knees.

"You haven't done that for a week." This is his way of telling me he wants me to do this every day.

"David, it gives me great pleasure and comfort to do this."

"Same for me, thank you."

Massaging his feet and legs is a new way for us to be present to each other and to give comfort.

I put clean socks on his feet and covered him with the prayer blanket that the ladies from Trinity Church had knitted for him. Sometime earlier this year when David was still able to attend church he was given the prayer blanket and I the shawl. We received them during Church and we were blessed and prayed for.

The aides come to take David to the bathroom. I go to the closet and dig out the quilt which is buried deep on the floor. The quilt is heavy and requires effort on my part to extricate. I fold it in thirds length wise, roll it up and place at the end of the bed.

"The Hospice nurse wants David's toes higher than his knees," I remind the aides.

Anna and Natalie transfer David to bed. Natalie pushes the quilt roll under his knees. Now his feet are lower than his knees but fortunately, Natalie places a pillow under his feet.

After lunch David is lying in his bed. We are lying together holding hands. Finally with privacy I'm able to address his request from last week.

"David, the other day you asked me to tell you the truth about what is happening... David you are dying... your death will come when the swelling on your brain stem increases."

"Speak English."

"David, picture what the brain looks like... the brain stem sits on top of your spinal column... the brain stem controls your voluntary muscles... We know that your voluntary muscles are affected...That's why you can no longer walk... feed yourself... and why it takes two people to transfer you from your chair to the toilet."

I wait for him to respond. I've been talking slowly with pauses to give him processing time.

"When the pressure on your brain stem increases... then the involuntary muscles to your heart will stop... Your heart and lungs will quit... and also your kidneys."

I continue to talk very slowly and with lots of pauses.

"David, the other possibility of the cause of death... comes from the blood clot in your left leg...

If the blood clot breaks up... then pieces could go to your heart and lungs and you will die... or the clot might go to your brain... causing a stroke."

Another long pause, "Nobody knows when you will die... it could be today... or several days from now... I will continue to be with you each day... I will massage your feet and put your socks on... I will feed you once a day... and I will lie with you and hold your hand."

"David, I love you and we will meet in Heaven."

"A-men," he sings.

Notes to myself:

1. Meet with Sharon, the Hospice social worker > help me know what I need to gather/do before his death.
2. Meet with Catherine and ask her to help me in planning the memorial service, she knows the liturgy so well.
3. Obituary.
4. What documents do I need? Such as our marriage certificate for Social Security.
5. Talk to Mike [my cousin] about helping file the legal stuff. Since I will be the widow, I can delegate someone to file or at least accompany and give me emotional support while I do what is required. It's the emotional support I need.
6. How long does the U of U medical school keep the corpse? How long before the ashes are returned?
7. Go this Friday to the Credit Union and close the account and open one under my name only and clear out the safe deposit box and switch it over to me.

11 September 3, 2011 Saturday

Yesterday, David ate a lot for breakfast according to Paula. The rest of the day he went downhill rapidly, no longer able to swallow, eat, or drink fluids. He was coughing a great deal.

Today when I came to see him at 1:30 pm the Hospice nurse came to assess him. Before she arrived a hospital bed had been set up.

David's kidneys are shutting down as well as his lungs. He coughs a great deal. The nurse says his heart will be the last to go. He could go tonight or tomorrow or it may take longer.

I sat next to him, holding his hand. *David squeezed my hand telling me he was glad that I was there.*

"David, I remember when we were still Catholics. Vatican II had taken place and the Mass was in English. Lay leaders were allowed to read the lessons. I was so proud of you for being a lay leader." *David squeezed my hand.*

"You were always spiritual. You led your parents, sister and brother back to the Church," *another squeeze.*

12 September 4, 2011 Sunday (Philip's birthday)

Marked decline by the time I arrived at noon. David's cough is gurgly and it sounds like his lungs are filled with fluid. The cough worsened by nightfall. He is being given Roxinall 1cc every hour. He seems comfortable, but no longer presses the hand that holds his.

Last night Paula and Philip stayed the night, taking turns sitting in the green winged recliner and holding his hand. The other slept on a camping pad with a pillow and coverings on the floor.

David is on oxygen @ 5 liters since yesterday. His saturation level is 81% and continues to fall.

At 12:30 pm, Father Don from Trinity came and visited with the family. We prayed the noon liturgy together.

As the afternoon progressed I stopped holding my husband's hand. I had learned from my hospice experience that continuing to hold the person's hand at the end can hold them back. [In 2013 as I read this, I realize I was in automatic mode, not taking in that all his organs were shutting down. Nothing would have kept him from passing.]

13   September 5, 2011 Monday (Labor Day)

David died this morning. Philip phoned me a few minutes before 8 am.

"Mom, Dad just took his last breath."

I hurried over. His hand was still warm.

Philip wanted his photo taken holding Dad's hand while his other hand gently touched the top of Dad's head. Paula took the photo.

"Dad, I love you and I'm going to miss you." Philip cried freely.

Philip's crying gave me the courage to hold David's hand while caressing his hair. Philip took the picture.

"David, I love you and your love I will carry in my heart forever. I will meet you in Heaven." For the first time since David was diagnosed with brain cancer, I cried, still swallowing my tears; though they splashed down my cheeks.

When the Hospice nurse arrived, Paula and Philip left the room. He was disconnected from his urine bag and the oxygen. I told her I wanted to help wash his body. I needed to be touching the body of my love for the last time.

The funeral director came in and wrapped his body and put it in a body bag and then on the cart. Philip, Paula, and I accompanied our dearly loved one out to the hearse. We went out the back way avoiding walking through the halls and lobby. The three of us returned through the lobby and there were several residents waiting for the procession to go by. They wanted to say their goodbyes.

Over the next three hours, we were busy clearing out his room. The green winged back recliner was moved to my apartment. His bed and dresser were given to an employee and his clothes went to Goodwill.

14 September 17, 2011 Saturday

My days are filled with settling affairs. Amidst the tasks, my mind goes blank. Frequently, I don't remember what I have done.

While my kitty Demetri settles in my lap, he no longer cuddles next to me when I'm sleeping and I wonder why.

15 September 24, 2011 Saturday

Settling affairs continues and I'm faced with limitations over what I can control.

The death certificate was delayed due to doctors disagreeing over who would sign. It took them ten days for the issue to be resolved.

In the meantime, I received a reimbursement check from long-term care insurance made out to David Brutz and the bank could not legally cash it. Last Monday I had gone to the insurance company's local office asking them to expedite having the check made out to me. Supposedly it was to have been done overnight.

16   September 26, 2011 Monday

Had to return to the social security office because I had received a notice informing me I would receive the amount of $843 each month; the regular amount I've been receiving. Fortunately the local office could pull up my awards notification which is yet to be mailed. I'm satisfied - the sum includes a widow's amount plus partial from my husband's SS totaling $1352.40. This is more than my husband's award and much less than our two combined which we had been receiving until his death.

And so it goes. Tomorrow I will return to the local office of my long-term insurance company and inquire about what is going on. I still need to go to the DMV for driver's licenses because mine does not reflect my current address.

Met Life Dental insurance mailed me two cards, both with David's name. I phoned and straightened it out. I'm in the midst of having dental work done. Last Thursday I had oral surgery. My eye tooth on the right side was pulled. It came out in pieces and pulled out a piece of the bone.

So the run-around goes on. When will everything be resolved?

I'm trying to establish a routine; hard to do while I'm settling affairs. The parts I know have to be in my routine are daily devotions, reformatting my book "Abuse-Survivors: Self-

Guided Retreat, a Memoir," eat properly, and exercise - which I do when I go to PT twice a week.

While socializing is helpful, I have a need to be alone much of the time, and there are moments when I just crawl in bed and sleep.

17   September 27, 2011 Tuesday

After doing physical therapy I trekked across town to the local office of the long-term care insurance company. Once again bureaucracy messes up. The local office called the national office. They had not received the check I had entrusted to the local office. It was suppose to have been faxed. But the national office had a record that the check had been issued and the September one is about to be released.

They require a copy of the death certificate. I'm confused about the various entities that were sending me a packet to fill out. Did I receive such a packet from long-term care insurance?

Now I'm waiting for them to mail a form which will enable them to make out the check in my name rather than the 'Estate of David Brutz.'

All bureaucracies have glitches in their systems, I suppose. But this one seems just unreasonable. I have to admit that I feel angry and would like to cuss them out, but I bury all those feelings.

18 December 31, 2011 Saturday

The last day of the year, I feel lost, adrift. I'm surprised that I'm asking, *"Who am I? What is my voice? I need to find my voice."*

Most of the affairs are settled now. I just received a check today for an IRA David had. Finally the long-term care insurance issues were settled. As frustrating as it was to go through, the process of getting things in order was at least something to hold onto in the changing current.

Now I'm adrift again. Where do I go? What do I do? The grief support group was not helpful, I'm sorry I kept attending. I resumed counseling which is what I need now. I'm crying a lot which is good.

Trying to figure out the business side of authoring and publishing, such as bookkeeping, publishing issues, and the electronic/digital details is very difficult. It is hard for me to focus and to think logically, seems like I'm in a fog much of the time.

Old survival skills from childhood are resurfacing. When I don't know how to approach something, I freeze. I want to hide, but I do make myself socialize by going to church and fellowship afterwards, to my Thursday morning coffee group in Old Town, and to Mustard Seed Dreams to knit. I've accepted invitations to go to lunch, breakfast, Christmas day dinner, and to movies. I joined church choir but left when my voice was wandering.

Funny that my singing voice is wandering, mirroring the life transition I'm going through. I need to find my voice.

I question the decisions I make. Was it a mistake to purchase snow tires for my car when four-season tires might have served me well and won't the snow tires decrease my fuel efficiency? Did I really need purchasing an I-Pod to listen to while I walk the treadmill?

I'm questioning everything I'm doing and not doing – this is all about insecurity. I feel so insecure. Am I living within my means? Will my funds last until I die? To whom can I turn to listen and talk to me through life? Who will companion me, walk alongside, and give me encouragement, feedback? These are the questions of the widow.

19 January 1, 2012 Sunday

Sources for inspiration came today at church from the lessons and we had a healing service.

As an adopted child of God, no longer a slave, God has sent the Spirit of his son into my heart. As his child, I am also his heir, (Galatians 4:4-7).

All that is 'good' is within me and I am to live that good in all that I do and am, therefore; away with negative framing. 'I'm lost, adrift' becomes instead 'I'm finding myself, I'm finding my moorings.' Further, 'I'm discovering a new world.'

The Blessing God gave to Moses for Aaron to bless the Israelites:

The Lord bless you and keep you;
The Lord make his face to shine upon you, and be gracious to you.
The Lord lift up his countenance upon you, and give you peace, (Numbers 7:22-27).

As far as my insecurities, I choose to focus on further developing, discovering how God's gift of my soul will reflect light into people's lives.

I went to a singles potluck in someone's home. Important lessons learned are one, I'm not ready, and two, the group is

LDS (Mormon); yes my age group, but not a good fit, not only because of religious affiliation, but there is no intellectual interchange and the main focus is eating. They meet weekly at restaurants. Most of the women weigh in excess of 300 lbs.

20 January 2, 2012 Monday

After gracefully leaving the social last night by saying it was too soon for me to be mingling, I phoned Paula. Megan answered, Paula was in the shower. I had Meg ask if I could come and hang out with them. Meg called back with a 'Yes.'

Delightful evening with my family, they were eating healthy, as they always do – fresh salad, and grilled chicken. I was able to eat with them. I had skipped the foods at the potluck.

At physical therapy this morning, I walked for 23 minutes on the treadmill with the sound aid of listening to Public Radio through my MP3 player. Paula set it up for me yesterday afternoon.

I've been mulling over my resolutions for this year, keeping in mind that they should be realistic.

1. Writing and publishing – schedule two days a week. Manage the business part on two days.
2. Exercise and fitness – stretching when I first wake up. Continue with PT 2x week. Increase walking time by 2 minutes a week.
3. Eating – return to my healthy pattern of eating and lose weight.
4. Social – return to HOPE, the cancer support group, attend adult education classes I'm registered for; visit Ray, a resident, at the care facility 2x week.

5. Continue with counseling.

I continue to have a long-term goal of being able to walk 4 miles. I would like to be able to go snow shooing and dare I dream about cross country skiing? Anyway, the physical therapy and increasing walking time lays the foundation for these goals to become realities.

21   January 9, 2012 Monday

Physical therapy goes well with greater ease in doing exercises, balance ball, arm cycle, leg press, and walking track. The balance platform continues to be a challenge. My knees hurt while tracing the infinity shape and when I step off, I have difficulty walking. Nonetheless, I'm encouraged.

When David was first in assisted living he was housed with the main population. He had his own room and he was assigned to a table for meals in the dining room. Ray was one of David's table mates.

My visit with Ray at the care facility went well. I took a copy of an illustrated "Aesop's Fables." My way to introduce the book, "Ray, I want to show you the illustrations. Would you like me to read the fable "The Bat, the Bramble bush and the Cormorant?"

I asked questions like, "What does their ship look like?" We loved it so we went onto "A Ladened Ass and a Horse." The illustration did not include the master. I asked, "What did the master's clothes look like?"

His answer, "Plaid."

We talked about the National Parks. Ray visited and camped at one. Asked about the bears in Yellowstone when he camped, "I ignore them."

22 January 15, 2012 Sunday (Second Sunday after Epiphany)

Hank, a lay leader, led us in Morning Prayer, I found his homily encouraging: "The Lord's call sometimes takes four times to hear. We need to be attentive that we don't fall into gluttony or other forms of waywardness."

I continue to work on my finances, consulting my State Farm agent and others. My financial advisor comments that it takes women longer to die than men, on the average of 3 ½ years. I'm still winding my path through long-term health insurance. My State Farm agent alerts me to the poor rating of the company I'm with.

I took my wedding band off. I'm no longer married. I am now a single woman. I'm feeling independent and stronger.

23   January 28, 2012 Saturday

The days go by quickly, although last Saturday was tough. Paula, my daughter, told me that they wouldn't be staying in the Pocatello area after the girls graduate from high school. She doesn't know where she and Tad will be going. She encourages me to do what is best for me. She also informed me that if I run out of money before I die, she will not help me. That was not all - she believes since I have had so many chronic illnesses that I won't live twenty more years anyway (when my IRA will run out). Neither was she encouraging about my writing, she thinks I shouldn't expect to come out ahead financially.

I felt like ice cold water had been thrown in my face. I felt unwanted and rejected, my over-riding feelings from childhood.

My wedding band is back on my finger. I need the comfort, reassurance, encouragement of my husband. He has faith in me, in my writing, in who I am.

Thursday when I went to Salt Lake for my medical appointment, I had a visit with Cousin Mike. He tells me that he and Julianne will be in Salt Lake for another three years. Again he invites me to relocate to where they will be. Told him if that is California, I wouldn't move there. If it is Oregon, I would consider.

What I've decided is to return to Cleveland Heights. Talked to Philip and asked if he would welcome me to return. "Of course!" was his immediate response. He encourages me to stay in Pocatello until the girls have left home, "Once the granddaughters are gone, they're gone. Now is the time to be around."

I long for a deep reconciliation with Paula. The deep rift hurts so much.

24   January 30, 2012 Monday

I cancelled going to an adult education class this morning and instead had productive contact with Create Space. As a result I was able to insert directions in the book manuscript regarding where the images go. Etc.

This afternoon, I worked on text for the back cover, the placement of the three endorsements, and the blurb about the author. Consulted my Iowa friend Kate about the wording and she helped me to tweak it.

My next task is to obtain a photo of myself, not clear yet how I will go about doing that.

25 January 31, 2012 Tuesday

Great News! Sandy, Dr. Karin Steven's assistant, phoned this morning to say that the Hep C virus has cleared my body!

26 February 2, 2012 Thursday

I attended Vera Thompson's funeral this morning. She was a member of the HOPE Cancer Support Group. She was a sassy woman. Dignified in her appearance; wearing hats, gloves, and jewelry. Vera was in her 90s and died from bone cancer.

The hospice chaplain's eulogy presented stories illustrating her strong-headed character, which he reframed as 'being passionate about life and in achieving goals.' "Towards the end she was able to move into peace with God, peace with herself, peace with her loved ones, and was able to let go and let God care for two members of her family who are not in good health. God could care better for them than she could."

I received in the mail a copy of Joan Didion's book "The Year of Magical Thinking," a memoir about the death of her husband and her grieving.

Didion begins her story with the death of her husband.

Oates begins her memoir "A Widow's Story, A Memoir" with the days leading up to her husband's death.

O'Kelly in "Chasing Daylight, How My Forthcoming Death Transformed My Life" begins his story of dying with his diagnosis.

Each author weaves in memories. Each describes scenes through their senses.

It makes sense to me to begin with the lead up to David's diagnosis – the month with the dramatic emergency of an MRI.

27 February 20, 2012 Monday

I created an author website, www.judybrutz.com.

Grateful for the insight and grace in healing my relationship with my daughter, still a ways to go, but we are making progress. I'm grateful for Paula's insights and openness.

Almost ready to file income tax, probably will do it tomorrow.

28 February 26, 2012 Sunday - First Sunday of Lent

Last night my granddaughter Julia and I went to the performance "Harmony: The Music of Life" by the Ambassadors from BYU-Rexburg. They did acrobatics, singing and dancing all simultaneously, truly amazing. It was good to share this experience with Julia. She is a young passionate ballet dancer.

I've received email that Create Space is sending me a bound copy of my book for proofing. I'm excited.

It is Lent. What does it mean to me this year? Retreat, Reconcile and Renew.

29   February 28, 2012 Tuesday

An AARP volunteer succeeded in filing my income tax today. Jean worked on my filing for more than two hours because it was complicated with deceased spouse and many kinds of deductions. Much to my relief and surprise I have sizable refunds coming from both federal and state governments.

30 March 3, 2012 Saturday

I completed the AARP'S Driver Training Program
yesterday. Helpful: how to scan; be attentive to all signs; 3-
second rule; imagine my route before starting; do flexibility
exercises and turn my body when I'm backing up. The
trainer recommends being a member of AAA in order to
receive maps and trip-ticks. But on the other hand, will I be
taking road trips?

31   March 5, 2012 Monday

The Proof copy of "Abuse Survivors: Self-Guided Retreat" arrived today. First run through, there are a lot of corrections to be made.

I received an acknowledgment from Council Gardens in Cleveland Heights that my name has been added to the waiting list. They advise that the wait will be about a year. I must phone them and discuss taking my name off the active list since I don't want to move to Cleveland Heights until my youngest granddaughter graduates from high school.

I feel like too much is going on.

32　March 11, 2012 Sunday - clocks set ahead

Longing to worship with Friends (Quakers), I traveled to Logan, Utah this morning and had the wonderful experience of watching the sun rise.

In thinking through my feelings and longings, I miss the deep spiritual connections that can happen in Friends Meetings for Worship and among individuals. I will not find this in the Episcopal Church. I will try to go to Logan whenever it seems feasible. It's a little less than a two hour trip one way through the mountains.

33 March 13, 2012 Tuesday

I'm no longer able to digest cheese; I became sick last night, vomiting and diarrhea splattered on the floor. I phoned Brenda at 9:15 pm (she does light housekeeping for me biweekly), fortunately she answered her phone and came over right away to clean up after me. I don't know what I would do without her.

Today is a new day, began to feel queasy, but drinking Ensure and an anti-nausea pill helped.

I received an email from Traci at FGC Friends General Conference (FGC) inviting me to look at the website for the Summer Gathering this year in New England. I've decided to register. It is costly but my tax refund will pay for most of it.

I long for fellowship/companionship with Quakers. The Society of Friends is my spiritual home and family. I know David would be pleased with my decision to go to the Gathering.

34   March 15, 2012 Thursday

I made airline reservations with Southwest Airlines for the trip to the FGC Gathering.

I'm feeling more relaxed and confident about my financial outlook.

Today's Lenten reading is comforting.

". . . and we get a vision of how we can be healed. By moving through our fear toward love itself, even when we feel like we may sink, we are close enough to feel God's loving hand holding us up." Rev. Becca Stevens, Lenten Meditations 2012, Episcopal Relief and Development

 * In reference to Peter's walking on the water and sinking

35 March 25, 2012 Sunday

I'm terribly sick again. I attended the "Progressive Dinner to Feed the 5,000." I thought I was careful in choosing which foods to eat, but there was a trigger food among the appetizers which I consumed at 6 pm. Not knowing that there was going to be a problem, I continued with the dinner, but at 8 pm when we were at St Anthony's for dessert, I felt sick and found the restroom and then the cycle started of vomiting. I drove home having to pull into the Office Max parking lot. I opened my door, leaned out and threw up on the pavement. It was raining and I wondered if the rain would wash the mess away or if the crows would come and have a feast. I continued to drive and had to pull over to the bike lane on Chubbuck Rd in front of Advantage-Plus Credit Union, again opening the door, leaning out and upchucking. I was anxious that the diarrhea would begin before I got into my apartment. Fortunately, I made it home without that happening. Barely.

I continued throwing up until 9:30 and then the overlap began. I sat on the toilet and held the waste basket. It was lined with a plastic bag. The diarrhea ended about midnight. Unlike previous such events, I sat in my recliner instead of going to bed. This saved soiling the carpet and floor. I placed a liner on the seat. I experienced severe chills, although when I was vomiting, I was sweating and felt hot. A cool cloth helped then.

Finally around 2 am I went to bed. Demetri, my kitty, stayed with me. Somehow he knows when I need him or at least I like to think that he does.

There is more to the weekend than being sick.

Yesterday afternoon, I had a wonderful grace-filled visit with Paula. We met in the lounge of her department at the University, being spring-break we had the whole place to ourselves.

I'm thankful to learn that Paula and Philip had visited by phone that morning. I was concerned that there was an estrangement between them. Paula pointed out that I had made an assumption and she affirmed to me that she does not hold grudges. It is good to get the "fuzzies" out of my brain. Our conversation focused on spirituality.

36   March 26, 2012 Monday

I received a phone call from Dr. Gilbert's office saying he wants to see me about the results of my labs. I wonder which values are out of range?

37 April 6, 2012, Good Friday

Difficult week in dealing with long-term insurance, will I ever be able to change agencies?

Then yesterday I ate food that triggered another gastrointestinal upset, need to have this taken care of.

I want to create a writing retreat for myself, thinking about how to do that at home as well as other places such as in my car, at a park, etc. To that end I cleared out and rearranged stuff in the apartment. I'm considering which books to get rid of.

I did manage to get rid of the air concentrator and oxygen tanks. My cardiologist says I don't need the Oxygen any longer, not even at night. I would like to be rid of the C-pap as well.

I registered for FGC Gathering 2012. I'm worried about food issues and traveling with C-pap, and laptop in addition to baggage. How will I manage?

38   April 7, 2012, Holy Saturday

Tonight I celebrated the Passover Seder with Temple Emanuel in Pocatello. Particularly meaningful to me this year is the *Dayeinu*.

"Our redemption from Egypt is but one example of the care God has shown us in our history. If God had done any one of these kindnesses, it would have been enough for us – in Hebrew Dayeinu. Dayeinu also reminds us that each of our lives is the cumulative result of many blessings, small and large."

Also meaningful is the introductory paragraph to *The Ten Plagues.*

"However, as we rejoice at our deliverance from slavery, we acknowledge that our freedom was hard-earned. We deeply regret that our freedom came at the cost of the Egyptians suffering, for we are human beings made in the image of God. Because of this, we pour out a drop of wine for each of the plagues as we recite them."

Is this the basis of Jesus' understanding of forgiveness? For me, Jesus is forever Jewish and his understanding of forgiveness came from his Jewish faith.

I particularly need to hear the *Dayeinu*. I want to remember that my life is the cumulative result of many blessings, small and large.

New birth with the Resurrection is to refocus on the cumulative result of many blessings both small and large rather than being overwhelmed with insecurity about the future.

Blessed be God.

39 April 10, 2012 Tuesday

I had a helpful talk with Paula last night about the wisdom of my traveling to New England because of my food issues and the management difficulties in traveling with suitcase, C-pap and laptop.

This morning I canceled my registration and feel relieved.

40   April 20, 2012 Friday

Tonight I canceled my air reservation with Southwest Airlines and they are refunding to my account.

This week I read *"Falling Upward, Spirituality for the Two Halves of Life"* by Richard Rohr.

"Stumbling over life's stumbling stones, you fail, you fall, you let go of the persona you created in the first half of life and 'Life – Fate – God – Grace – Mystery' gets you to change, to let go in order to go on the further and larger journey. You go through necessary suffering which is a crucible. One experiences daily dying even while trying to avoid dying."

This is a valuable book. It reminds me of Joyce Rupp's book which I'm now re-reading, "Walking in a Relaxed Manner, Life Lessons on the Camino."

Progress. I completed another round of proofreading for my book today and talked to the coordinator of my design team. Next week I will check with them to make sure the change file was uploaded properly.

All-in-all this has been an energized and blessed week.

Thank you, Lord.

41   April 23, 2012 Monday

Saturday I went to the ballet of Cinderella. Julia danced as one of the Royal friends and of course she did superbly. After seeing Walt Disney's Cinderella, the ballet seems slow. Part way through the performance Megan rested her head on my shoulder – a treasured moment.

Prior to the ballet I went to the monthly writers group which meets at Marshall Public Library. We had a guest who led us in a writing exercise. **A poem popped out for me.**

2Nothing was the same
Now that it was twilight.
His lips didn't move
Was he still breathing?
I know he died this morning
But how do I really know?
Will he come through the door in the dark?
And climb in beside me? Hold me close?

It is 11:30 and I'm so very tired, off to bed I go. In the morning, I have an 8 am appointment to have an ultrasound of my gallbladder.

42   April 26, 2012 Thursday

I'm thankful to have received a report of my ultrasound and I'll take it with me to my appointment with Dr. Gilbert. The report says I have a large gallstone. I asked to be referred to my general surgeon, Dr. Harmon, who now has his practice in Burley, Idaho.

Paula wants to drive me to my surgery appointment and bring me home. We discussed which dates would work for her. I'm so thankful she wants to be with me.

43   May 3, 2012 Thursday

I was knocked for a loop at the dentist's - a front tooth has to be pulled and is scheduled for 4:45 pm tomorrow. I'll phone Dr. Harmon to inform him and see if the gallbladder surgery will need to be postponed.

Okay, we're good to go, no need to delay the surgery, just need to remember to stop taking Pradaxa.

When faced with the decision to pull the tooth, I made the decision quickly and confidently, but emotionally, I feel disoriented and anxious about my schedule for the next couple of days. I became anxious about Paula's tight schedule. Childhood abuse and neglect issues are stirred up about being in the way and not being able to do what I was expected to do and then consequently being rejected or judged in some way. One such event happened when I was 10 years old.

It was Mother's birthday and I was begging her not to go out that evening. Every night, it seemed, she went out to a lounge, without my step-father, and came home late or not at all. I had baked a birthday cake, but she would not acknowledge either me or the birthday cake. She continued to put on her eye makeup. I was crying and so upset that I smashed the cake on the floor and she left without saying a word.

Why does this stuff still pop up?

Spiritually I'm trying to trust God completely, but how easily I fail.

44 May 10, 2012 Thursday

I had surgery this morning to remove my gallbladder - went well. Dr. Harmon is attentive, friendly, and interactive.

Paula is with me, attentive, caring, and loving. Her love overcomes my fears about being abandoned.

Thank you, Lord.

45 May 15, 2012 Tuesday

I voted in the Primary today and visited with Jennifer, an acquaintance, bringing her up to date. Tears flowed about David. We always voted together including the smallest elections.

David, I miss you – rock tough and soft feelings. Each time I see TV shows, I think of you. You would be sitting there in the cherry rocker intently watching, apron tied around your neck to protect you from spilling. You would be eating the oatmeal left over from the morning. You would hold the pan and eat from it. Oh, my Love.

46   May 17, 2012 Thursday

David, I want your comfort tonight. So much is going on.

How do I keep it altogether?

47　May 26, 2012 Saturday

I went with Billie, a woman friend from church, to Poky Free Bikes. I donated $25 for an old classic Schwinn. They weren't able to fit tires, but they did raise the handle bars, put on an extra reflector and a wire pannier. We went to a sports store where they repair bikes. They were able to order from a catalogue tubes and tires. I purchased a handle bar mirror. They are keeping the bike until the tires come in.

Billie asked me what I'm going to name the bike. I've never done that before, but think it's a good idea. "Courage," I told her.

"Courage" is green and a cruiser. It will be a while before I will try riding it. I won't ride until I get the "go ahead" from Richard, my physical therapist. I'll probably ride when I'm able to cycle on the stationary for two miles and however many minutes that will take (16?). Also I want to be able to do greater challenges on the Bosu Balance Ball or whatever balancing challenge comes next. We'll see.

Also, I asked Billie if she would accompany me to Coeur d'Alene to ride the special bike trail there. I'm about the age Billie's mother would be. Her mom died when Billie was still in her teens.

Philip phoned. He has four tickets to the Indian Baseball Game on September 1st. It is time to make plane reservations to arrive a couple of days in advance. We will be celebrating Philip's 50th birthday and it will be the first anniversary of David's death.

I told Philip about my bicycle riding goal. He was speechless, dumb-founded and totally silent. He hasn't seen me for nine months and has no idea how well I am able to walk, balance and have stamina. He will be surprised when he sees me. I hope I'm riding "Courage" by then.

48   May 29, 2012 Tuesday

Talked to Philip yesterday, I called. He was at his friend's Memorial Day Picnic. Philip says that my granddaughter Heather and her boyfriend will be home for Labor Day Weekend.

I told Philip about Richard advancing my balancing exercise to alternating standing on one leg one minute at a time on the Bosu Balance Ball. Philip was impressed, said he wouldn't be able to do that.

Today I lifted a 20 lb box of kitty litter that is definitely my limit. Pleased to know what my upper limit is and indicates how much further I hope to strengthen in order to lift 50 lb.

49 July 24, 2012 Saturday

Last night I walked the "Memorial Walk" for David at the Pocatello Relay for Life. My friends, Audrey, Nancy, and Lynda accompanied me. By email I had sent out a request to our Thursday morning coffee group which meets in Old Town that I need companions.

During the week there was a heat wave sending temps to 103 degrees. Friday the temperature slowly declined as cloud cover moved in. By the time Audrey and Nancy picked me up, around 9 pm, rain began to hesitantly sprinkle.

I located the HOPE support group members sitting in lawn chairs under a shade canopy. Allan guided me to the luminary he had made for David.

Shortly after 10 pm the stadium lights were shut off and the names of the cancer survivors who died during the past year were read.

"Did you hear David's name?" my companions queried, but I hadn't.

We walked for as long as I could which was forty minutes.

I felt numb, I miss him so much. I wore the last hat that was knitted for him. Paula had made it for her Dad and he wore it 24-7 the last several weeks he lived. I also wore one of the vests he had us purchase at Fred Meyers. He was well then and had taken the initiative to go looking for vests for me.

Last night I wore the lavender-purple one. The hat and vest both comforted and shielded me from the rain that was off and on. I carried a luminous stick with a heart at the tip that Debbie gave me when I visited the HOPE canopy.

I also wore a pair of running shoes I purchased yesterday morning, knowing I needed good foot gear for the occasion. The day before, I had walked 35 minutes at OK Park wearing my LL Bean leather sandals. The ridge under the toes made the underside of the right third toe sore.

Why all this attention to the physical as I write? Because I miss David's physical presence, his walking beside me holding hands.

I recall when we drove to the Walden Pond in autumn weather in 1961. We took each other's hands and married each other then and there. That December the priest officially married us in the Byzantine Catholic Church.

Now I want his cremains returned to me. His cadaver is in some building at Idaho State University being used by students to study anatomy. Paula tells me that the ashes won't be returned until 2017, five years from now. I must have been told this at the time of his death but I was in such a blank, I don't recall what I was told.

I'm faced with the reality that I am planning to return to Cleveland Heights after Julia graduates from high school.

Last night I began to ponder remaining in Pocatello until his ashes are returned to me and then going with Philip and Paula to Yellowstone and scattering them.

The logistics of my return move to Cleveland Heights are troublesome. Thankfully I don't have to figure that out at this time.

"Logistics" is a good term for the emotional state I'm in these days. I'm having difficulties figuring out and doing the connective work with my computers, digital devices, and wifi modem so I can do what I want with my writing.

How do I proceed with moving forward when I'm in a state of limbo?

50   July 14, 2012 Saturday

Last night I walked the "Memorial Walk" for David at the Pocatello Relay for Life. My friends, Audrey, Nancy, and Lynda accompanied me. By email I had sent out a request to our Thursday morning group that meets in Old town "I need companions."

During the week there was a heat wave temps to 103 degrees. Friday the temperature slowly declined as cloud cover moved in. By the time Audrey picked me up around 9 pm, rain began to hesitantly sprinkle.

I located the HOPE support group members sitting in lawn chairs under a shade canopy. Allan guided me to the luminary he had made for David.

Shortly after 10 pm the stadium lights were shut off and the names of the cancer survivors who died during the past year were read.

"Did you hear David's name?" my companions asked, but I hadn't.

We walked for as long as I could which was forty minutes.

I felt numb, I miss him so much. I wore the last hat that was knitted for him. Paula had made it for her dad and he wore it 24-7 the last several weeks he lived. I also wore one of the vests he had us purchase at Fred Meyers. He was well then and had taken the initiative to go looking for vests for me.

Last night I wore the lavender-purple one. The hat and vest both comforted and shielded me from the rain that was off and on. I carried a luminous stick with a heart at the tip that Debbie gave me when I visited the HOPE canopy.

I also wore a pair of running shoes I purchased yesterday morning, knowing I needed good foot gear for the occasion. The day before, I had walked 35 minutes at OK Park wearing LL Bean leather sandals. The ridge under the toes made the underside of the right toe sore.

Why all this attention to the physical as I write? Because I miss David's physical presence, his walking beside me holding hands.

I recall when we drove to the Walden Pond in autumn weather in 1961. We took each other's hands and married each other then and there. That December the priest officially married us in the Byzantine Catholic Church.

Now I want his cremains returned to me. His cadaver is in some building at Idaho State University being used by students in their anatomy studies. Paula tells me that the ashes won't be returned until 2017, five years from now. I must have been told this at the time of his death but I was in such a blank, I don't recall what was said.

I'm faced with the reality that I am planning to return to Cleveland Heights after Julia graduated from high school.

Last night I began to ponder remaining in Pocatello until the ashes are returned to me and then with Philip and Paula and other family members going to Yellowstone and scattering them where it is permitted.

The logistics of my return move to Cleveland Heights are troublesome. Thankfully I don't have to figure that out at this time.

"Logistics" is a good term for the emotional state I'm in these days. I'm having difficulties figuring out and doing the connective work with my computers, digital devices and wifi modem so I can do what I want with my writing.

How do I proceed with moving forward when I'm in a state of limbo?

51 July 21, 2012 Saturday

I'm back on Lexapro and fortunately FDA approved a generic form in March of this year. Dr. Gilbert happily wrote me a prescription. I'm doing well so I won't see him for another six months.

It occurs to me that it would be wise to set goals to help me be more focused. Otherwise I will reach the end of my life and be disappointed that I was lackadaisical. In other words, I'm making a "**bucket list**."

Relationships:

- Resolve relationship issues keeping in mind to change the things I can change and not to take on the blame for those things I cannot change.
- Be social by inviting people to do things with me. Don't isolate.
- Express gratitude.

Fitness:

- Walk
- Bike
- Exercise
- Low carb and lactose free diet

Home-Care:

- Do most everything myself
- Have housekeeper come biweekly

Small Business:

- Learn skill sets or contract out tasks
- Develop my business as author
- Self-publish – prayers, widowing, peace

Breathing:

- Use my c-pap machine

Service: Be careful not to become overly involved

- Lead small group(s) at church
- Be involved in First Friday Art Walk at church
- Become a member of Pastoral Care Partners
- Teach adult education classes in the community

Spirituality:

- Worship
- Spiritual disciplines

Relocate: Return to Ohio in 4-5 years.

Live as though this is my last year.

Be organized.

Be Grateful.

52   July 30, 2012 Monday

The homily yesterday focused on 'wants' vs. 'needs.' I have to ask myself "Are my goals 'wants' or 'needs'?" I don't know.

My prayer is, *"Help me to touch peoples' lives, Lord, according to your will. Guide me each day. Help me to be focused and organized."*

We, members of the HOPE support group, have been asked to have focused check-ins and to express our emotions about our state of being.

In a few minutes, I enter the HOPE meeting room. How am I?

I miss David, I am depressed and anxious. While I'm socially involved and accomplish things, I tend to vegetate 4-6 hours a day.

My doctor has placed me on generic Lexapro and I know that will help.

Good news, I go to Salt Lake tomorrow to see my liver doctor. I expect to be discharged. I look forward to being with two cousins for a couple of days.

53   August 1, 2012 Wednesday

Dr. Kerin Stevens discharged me. The Hep C has been cured. I'll miss my visits with her because she is a supportive and caring person. I need that with David gone. She inquired about what I'm doing. I gave her one of my promotional cards for my book "Abuse Survivors: Self-Guided Retreat." She asked me for as many cards as I could give her for both patients and the providers who are always looking for resources. I'm encouraged by her enthusiastic response.

On Monday night at the HOPE meeting, the social worker led us in a discussion of "the tyranny of being positive." I came away with the thought to give myself some slack for vegging out each day for a period of time. Instead of this being "negative," I'm recharging my batteries by sleeping and "just" being quiet and this is all part of my grieving.

Good day yesterday with cousins Mike and Julianne. We looked through the one photo album Mike has from his parents' early part of their marriage. We went to lunch and then to the Pagoda Earrings so I could buy a pair with stainless steel posts.

Last night I stayed at La Quinta Hotel, what an extremely comfortable bed, I would gladly return. I wish my bed was as good.

I watched the Olympics in my room. Michael Phelps won his 19th medal in his team's relay and the USA women's gymnastics team won gold.

54 August 3, 2012 Friday – Monastery of the Ascension, Jerome, Idaho

EfM Training for Mentors (Education for Ministry)

Months ago, don't remember exactly when it was, Diane Paulson asked me to consider taking training with her to become mentors for EfM.

I'm here at the Jerome Monastery for the 18 hour training. I am surprised about being here - don't know what this program is. Do I accept the apparent call?

I have the gifts, training and experience to do mentoring. I use theological reflection, and I seek the deeper spirituality which can be found through the Bible. I long for the community and worship that EfM group members create. Going through the four year program as a mentor would afford me a means to plug into the EfM program in Cleveland. I would be part of a community rich in interconnectedness and I would have purpose.

Yes, I accept the call.

What are the implications for my writing?

What are my priorities?

55 August 13, 2012

Priorities: I had been exploring becoming a Personal Historian, but am dropping that because my own writing comes first. I'm resigning from being Precinct Captain because I'm too introverted to do the door-to-door and phone canvassing. The stress of doing extroverted tasks results in my shutting down and becoming highly anxious.

"Shutting down," also a term for vegging out, I veg out for four to six hours at a time. Yes, I am drained of energy, a real introvert, but it is also grief. I have many ways of denying that I am grieving.

Today I requested Dr. Gilbert to again place me on Buspar or whatever its proper name is. Being on a SSI and an anti-anxiety med will help balance my neurochemical functioning.

Tonight the HOPE support group was particularly helpful. We had our break-out group for supporters and our social worker asked "Describe your style of coping" and later, "How do you know when there is closure?" I silently wondered if one of my ways of coping is "disassociating."

Through the discussion tonight I came to the epiphany that the gift of being assigned to mentor an EfM group is that I have a way of being anchored when I turn inward.

In the last week I was reminded of the Meyers Briggs mapping of personality traits. My profile characteristics are INFJ. This is helping to understand once again that I am an Introvert (very clear), N intuitive (very clear), F feeling (clear), and J plan ahead (clear). The J factor is strength to balance the INF characteristics. I'm blessed.

I can use the J trait starting now by studying the EfM "Common Lessons and Supporting Materials" which is over 600 pages. This way I will be prepared by January when our group will hopefully start.

Thank you Lord.

56   August 14, 2012 Tuesday

No vegging out today, after PT this morning I took a ride north on Yellowstone Rd. and arrived at Fort Hall where I turned around and followed various roads to see the land, homes, and crops. It was like doing labyrinth by car, the center of the labyrinth being home.

On Sunday afternoon I took a similar drive going north on Hawthorne Rd., then west on Reservation Rd. That labyrinth trip started at Trinity Church and again the circuitous route centered at home.

My approach is to be open to the experience. This is one of the ways I walk the labyrinth. Be open to the experience.

What did I experience - Movement, exploration of the unknown, a sense of the Presence being with me, and a sense of being loved. Julian of Norwich's words come to mind, *"All will be well, and all matter of things will be well again."*

For lunch I experimented making a small buckwheat pancake, substituting part of the 1/3 cup buckwheat mix with almond flour to reduce carbs and to increase the protein. Delicious.

Then I turned to studying the Common Lessons and supporting materials of EfM as well as lesson plans from the students' material. I'm trying to grasp hold of the broad-sweep and then pickup on details, very much like my going through special museum exhibitions. I walk through to get a feel for the whole and then return to view specifics, including reading or listening to the audio guide.

The EfM material is challenging, even overwhelming. It is graduate level theological studies. On the surface the material appears to be solely academic, but the exercises actually integrate the whole person in relation to group members and with God, koionea is created, quite remarkable.

Thank you for this day. I'm blessed.

57 August 17, 2012 Friday – Paula's Home

I'm so pleased to be asked to house and dog-sit for my family. Ella and Ivan are comfortable with me and I love them. Crookie is nowhere to be seen. Ella and Ivan are black labs and Crookie is an orange tabby.

The haze from all the fires in Idaho makes for poor air quality. I find I cannot do activities outside because I get a sore throat and am coughing up mucous. Fortunately, I'm not developing bronchitis, at least so far. Dr. Gilbert is diagnosing me with asthma instead of chronic bronchitis.

I registered on-line for the Bishop's retreat in October. It will be at the monastery in Jerome, love that place.

This morning I worked out at PT. I always feel so good afterwards. I've lost 3 lbs in the last 10 days thanks to being stricter with lower carbs, higher protein and an increase in oil.

My mental health has improved with taking generic Lexapro and Buspar. Thankfully my insurance pays for these meds.

I have a couple of weeks before traveling to Cleveland Heights. I plan on pushing to make progress on family history.

My book ought to be up on Kindle any day. I need to develop a marketing strategy.

Wednesday night Diane Paulson and I met with the Vestry, a group of church members who manage the church. They are excited about the two of us being accredited to mentor EfM. Also, I shared with vestry the news about my book being published. Senior Warden is having the church secretary order copies for our library. I'm asking Father Don to bless the ministry of my book at worship this coming Sunday.

58 August 20, 2012 Monday

Yesterday, Holy Eucharist worship was held in the courtyard with Rev. Don Paulson officiating. After the blessing of the prayer shawls, he had me come forward with a copy of my book "Abuse Survivors: Self-Guided Retreat, a Memoir of Healing." He held the book up so everyone could see the cover and said a few words about it and why it is an important book and ministry.

Don had me face him and we held the book together with the book being horizontal and the cover in the reading position for him. With his left hand he made the sign of the cross three times in the same manner that he consecrates the bread. Don spoke but I don't remember what he said. Everyone was moved to a deep silence.

During the homily Don gave instruction on the difference between 'Bio' and 'Zoe.' Bio gives food for the flesh while Zoe gives eternal life, life of the Spirit. By consecrating the ministry of my book and my special ministry through it, the gift of life is Zoe.

At coffee time, a few people came up to congratulate me and to take a look at the book. I feel humbled and thankful.

59   August 21, 2012 Tuesday

To my joy, Paula phoned this evening and asked if I would like to stay with Megan over this coming weekend while the rest of the family goes to Montana. Tara, the puppy, will be at home and Megan will run her. I will drive Megan to and from work.

60 August 26, 2012 Sunday

This has been a wonderful weekend. Staying overnight with Megan and parts of each day has been a blessing. The dogs were a handful in a pleasant way. I was able to train Tara to stay away from Crookie, the old orange tiger cat. Ella and Tara play endlessly, each trying to take the red Kong from the other and each displaying alpha status by humping. Ella finally established her dominance for the day at least, shown by Tara lying down on her back. Tara also challenges Ivan to play. He barks at her. He doesn't want to be bothered as old as he is – 12 years old, I think.

61   August 30, 2012 Thursday – Cleveland Heights, Ohio

Long hours of travel, I got up at 1 am Mountain Time this morning and arrived in Cleveland 6:30 pm Central Time. I don't know why I was so anxious the last few days, am I always like this before a trip?

Philip picked me up at the airport and is impressed with how much fitter I am. He says, "It is quite striking the difference from last year. You even walk faster."

Philip drove me through the grounds of Council Gardens. The grounds are beautiful. Philip suggests that his friend Peter could show me around including his apartment. We measured the distance between Council Gardens and Philip's home and it is 2 miles; nice walking distance.

My relationship with Philip is comfortable. He is open about his feelings and thoughts and engages in personal conversation with me.

I look forward to living in Cleveland Heights again. It is a better fit than Pocatello because of the diversity and progressive views.

I would move now except that I wish to stay four more years in Pocatello in order to be there while Megan and Julia are still in high school and also to complete the four year cycle of mentoring EfM. Hopefully I will be able to be involved in the EfM program in Cleveland.

62   September 2, 2012 Sunday – Cleveland Heights, Ohio

Kathy, an old friend, picked me up this morning and dropped me off at Quaker Meeting. From a distance I didn't recognize her. Her hair is white, long to her waist, and held in a pony tail at the nape of her neck. She wore jeans and a tee shirt. Up close her face is recognizable. Years ago, Kathy had shoulder length dark hair, never pulled back and she wore professional clothing.

Meeting attendance was small due to the Labor Day Weekend. The atmosphere was comfortable, relaxed and open in contrast to what I experienced a few years ago when I came from Iowa for a visit with family. Then the pocket doors to the meeting room were closed to keep late comers from walking in. Friends had to wait in the hall until the children were released to go to First Day School. The feeling was restrictive, not welcoming and certainly not friendly.

I visited with old friends. Marty warmly hugged me. Vickie came up and neither of us recognized the other because of our aging. I identified Gerry, but he didn't recognize me.

Chris was not in the meeting when I attended decades ago. He is now the clerk and has been with Cleveland Meeting for ten years. He is gentle, open and friendly. He invited volunteers for the day to clean up after the soup meal. No one volunteered.

"You're each on your own to clean up." He requested that someone lock up the Meeting House and someone did volunteer. Chris gave me a lift to Philip's.

Chris tells me that the meeting has 'reached clearness' about finding a suitable place to meet 'as way opens' and at that time they expect to sell the Meeting House. I miss being with Friends (Quakers) and the expressions we use about our decision making process. At the same time I miss being with Trinity Episcopal friends and the liturgy.

Chris informs me of recent deaths within the last couple of years, Kathy and Ted Wood, and Betsy Walker. Chris will mail me a new Meeting Directory when it is completed.

Philip's birthday gathering today was a joy. Six family members came and were joined by several of Philip and Ruth's friends - Liz and William, Robin, Holly and Brad, and their two year old, Stella.

The menu included Philip's favorite foods – chicken paprikash and Kalula cake. Long green beans from the garden were fresh and delicious. Hanna, Philip's mother-in-law, contributed a German dish which consists of small finger-nail length pasta stir fried in butter and browned onion. Philip and Ruth's daughters, Heather and Katharine made the Kalula cake; absolutely heavenly. Philip and Ruth's friend Holly made home-made vanilla ice cream and someone brought a watermelon. Wine, beer, and ice water were available.

I'm struck with how attentive, thoughtful, and caring Philip is to me – such as putting in two window air conditioners and switching them on to reduce the humidity, helping me with my laundry, as well as sitting next to me.

Philip phoned his friend Peter who lives in Council Gardens. Peter moved there maybe 13 years ago on disability. He is now around sixty years old. Peter invites Philip, Hanna and me over for tomorrow around noon to give us a tour and to see his apartment.

63 September 3, 2012 Labor Day – Cleveland Heights

Peter took us to his apartment before showing us around. His apartment is about the same size as mine (a plus), but no hookups for laundry (a minus). The residents are diverse both racially and ethnically, predominantly Jewish (diversity is a plus). The grounds are beautiful with gardens of various kinds – vegetables, fruit, flowers, and lots of trees (plus). It is located in Cleveland Heights (a plus); having the senior center down the street (a plus); being two miles from Philip (triple plus); and being close to University Circle (a plus). Another plus is the security found in a senior community.

The process of moving is anxiety producing – the logistics. Leaving Trinity parish will be a loss. Right now I'm thinking of selling all my furniture and appliances but not my bookcases and books.

In some ways, I would like to move now. Holding me back is my wanting to be around my two youngest granddaughters until they both leave home. I want to deepen and enrich my relationship with them. Also, I want to go through the full four year EfM cycle.

What will I do with my religious affiliation? Do I want to continue being affiliated and connected with the Friends (Quakers)? I would like to carry out dual affiliation, but how? Am I a chameleon?

64   September 4, 2012 Tuesday – Cleveland Heights and Philip's 50th birthday

A treat on Philip's birthday; he arranged for Hanna and me to have behind-the-scenes tour of the Cleveland Museum of Art. Mary, the oversight administrator for the whole museum, took us through an exhibit being prepared for Gallery One. It is an educational, interactive experience for children, emphasizing shapes, colors, subjects, and themes.

Philip has been with the Museum for six years. I'm so proud of his accomplishments as head mounter. He works with the conservators in textiles, glass, paper, photos, paintings, statues, jewelry, and on-and-on.

A couple of nights ago Philip declared that he is an atheist as well as Heather and Katharine, his daughters.

"You follow in the footsteps of your great grandfather."

"And my grandmother as well."

My thought, each person finds where they are comfortable. I'm feeling saddened if not bordering on grieved. What is, is.

65   September 5, 2012 Wednesday – Cleveland Heights, Ohio

One Year Anniversary

Dear David,

One year since you breathed your last and I still find myself each day saying out loud, "David, help me."

66 September 8, 2012 Saturday – Pittsburgh

Philip and I drove to Pittsburgh to visit David's mother and Philip's grandmother, Kate, who is wheelchair bound. It was startling to see her face, puffier now since she has gained a little weight and needed to. With her glasses off, I thought I was looking at David when he was wheelchair bound and his face was puffy from being on steroids. My heart was pulled. I wondered how he could be dead.

Next month Kate will be 97 years old. She reminded me that David had said many times before he became ill that he was going to live as long or longer than she.

Kate thinks of David everyday and misses his frequent phone calls and his coming to visit her. She thought it was too much for him to come by bus across the country to see her.

When we were at the restaurant I was further startled when Kate would stare blankly and not follow the discussion. I was seeing David when he could no longer keep pace, couldn't understand the words. Their eyes are the same color which I had not noticed previously. The difference in their blank stare is that when we addressed Kate she immediately perked up and engaged. Her mind is sharp. Her memory is excellent. In fact, she could recall names before the rest of us did.

Another recollection she had when we were still in her room at Canteberry was how David would climb the stairs instead of taking the elevator and then he would do pushups on her floor. Yes, very David – his fitness program.

David has the gentleness, kindness, patience and loyalty of his mom. He was strongly influenced by her.

Ellen, my sister-in-law's daughter, calls me "Aunt Judy." I've been a poor, inactive aunt. I have not connected with being an aunt. Hopefully, it is not too late. I've got to get with it. I do want to be connected to family and it is up to me to establish those connections.

67   September 13, 2012 Thursday – Pocatello

Today I registered for a four week class on how to use my Canon Digital camera. Between mine and David's illnesses and his dying, I haven't used the camera since we took the Alaska cruise. I've forgotten how to use it.

I charged the camera battery this afternoon in time for the first session at the Art Supply Center of Pocatello on Center Street across from Maag's Pharmacy.

A year anniversary since David dies and I am ready to use the camera. Richard Albright, our teacher, advised me to take off the protective rubber case allowing the camera to be more easily used. David in his safety and protective mode insisted that we use the protective covering. Now I am able to make my own choices about whether I use protective gear or not.

 I was surprised to learn that the memory card is filled and it has 2 GB capacity. Downloading the data onto the simple drive I will be able to view all the photos David and I took together. This takes my breath away. I will be viewing snap shots of our lives since we've been in Pocatello. Maybe this will feel like I can let go of wanting the cremains returned to me before the five years are up.

***

Memories from Our Alaska Cruise

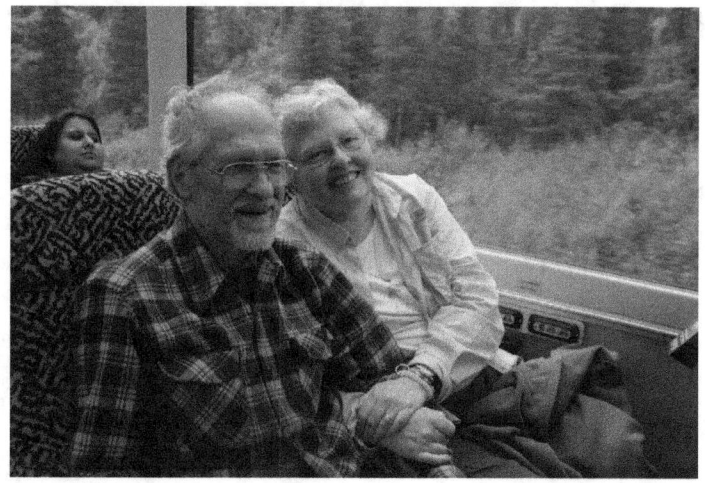

Sorting through the digital images from our Alaska trip, I chose a photo of David and me sitting together on an excursion train on its way to Denali National Park. David sitting on the aisle, I next to the window, our arms intertwined, holding hands. The picture emanates light and joy.

It was David who brought up the idea of taking a cruise. I was more than a little dumbfounded. We had been frugal all our married life. Spending thousands of dollars on such a luxury seemed extreme. He convinced me.

"We must go while you still can. This may be the last year you will be able to go."

As I look back, the whole situation is remarkable. I was not well. It was thought that I had Parkinson's and I was the one

139

declining rapidly. We believed that I would be the first to go, leaving David to cope without me. David was thinking of me, loving me, wanting me to have a wonderful, beautiful, and once-in-a-life time adventure.

"How about Hawaii?" David asked.

"I would rather go to Alaska."

We didn't say what was on our minds, but we were really dealing with a bucket list for me.

Lots of memories flooded me as I looked at the digital photos. I decided to change my cover photo also. It shows runoff from a glacier feeding a lake below. This photo I downloaded from Google images. So magnificent.

One of the neatest thrills I had when we were in Denali was the last day we were there, a clear blue sky without clouds.

David wasn't one to go in airplanes ever. For instance, when I went to visit my mother in San Francisco, I would fly from Iowa and David would take the Greyhound bus meeting me at my mother's apartment. On the last day in Denali, David was pleased for me to take a puddle jumper without him.

The little plane flew around Denali Peak and all five of us passengers landed on a glacier feeding off the peak. AND I walked on the glacier ice with the aid of my cane which has a crampon for such conditions. This was extraordinary considering that I had been getting around on an electric scooter even on the ship. The sky was so blue. There were no clouds. There was some kind of a little wooden structure up on a crag. Who could have built it? And what was its purpose?

It was hard to believe that I was on this glacier and that as we flew around in a tiny plane that the sky was so clear we were able to see the mountain top. I was told this is rare. I took many photos both from the plane and walking on the glacier.

68   September 23, 2012 Saturday

Even though I'm doing many things and am socializing, I'm washed through with sadness. My inclination is to withdraw, to be alone, and so I have cutback, is it enough?

69 September 24, 2012 Sunday

Eucharistic service – worship lifted me and fills me with hope, with a glimmer of confidence in my gifts and blessings. Don's sermon was on women-wisdom (Proverbs 31:10-31) and on being peaceable, gentle, willing to yield, and to be full of mercy (James 3:17). Don rendered the meaning of "fear of the Lord" – not to be taken literally, rather to have awe, loyalty, and respect for God.

I resigned from the First Friday Art Walk team, but did give Barbara the suggestion of featuring the artist George Wise. I feel a sense of relief with resigning.

I talked with Diane Paulson. She helped me see that I could go ahead and sign up to teach a writing class with adult education and then if facilitating an EfM group is too demanding, then I can cancel the writing class. This is an excellent resolution and once again I feel relieved.

70 September 26, 2012 Wednesday

I believe that God uses our gifts to bring love and healing into the world.

"Let love be genuine, reject evil, hold fast to what is good, love one another with mutual affection, do not lack in zeal, be ardent in spirit. Serve the Lord. Rejoice in hope, be patient in suffering, persevere in prayer. Extend hospitality to strangers." Romans 12:9-13

"We are to use our different gifts in accordance with the grace that God has given us. . .Whoever shares with others should do it generously." Romans 12:6, 8

71   October 1, 2012 Monday

Each day is a mixture of being active and being paralyzed by fear and anxiety.

72 October 12, 2012 Friday

Even though I've been busy taking classes and going on retreat, underneath I'm deeply grieving. I haven't fully accepted that David is completely dead and gone. Still each day I call out *"David, help me."* And even when I was on retreat and asked to raise our fingers to indicate how many of the three people we had identified as being important in forming who we are, I only raised two fingers, not acknowledging that David had died!

When I'm outside my apartment, I'm very good at covering or rather keeping private my inner state. At home my grief is experienced as despair, as in not wanting to do anything, of wanting to give up. What saves me is knowing that David wants me to have a satisfying life.

God with me, Amen.

The retreat "Praying in Color" with Sybil MacBeth is opening nonverbal ways of praying involving doodling. I've been helped so much and think my praying in this manner makes me aware of my inner condition. My prayer journal for this morning is revealing.

"Do not let your hearts be troubled and do not be afraid."
John 14:27

Holding my prayerful feelings and words I doodle, coloring God's energy infusing my creation on paper.

146

This afternoon an insight, *Put aside your writing the book. It is not time.* I've been working on my widowing book.

73 October 20, 2012 Saturday

The grief is a deep depression. Praying through drawing is helping me, insights and openings occur.

I'm seeking inspiration on my next writing project, what will it be?

EfM is coming up. I will consult with Diane on having registrants fill out the forms and move on ordering the manuals. It seems I'm to take the administrative lead on this since Diane is working full-time and in fact, she asked me to.

74   October 23, 2012 Tuesday

My new prayer practice is remarkably effective in connecting me with God when I stop being highly verbal. I pray for others. I pray scripture. I have a way to discern spiritual guidance.

I'm calmer, more peaceful. My breath prayer is *"Loving God, comfort and guide me."* The depression-grief has lifted.

My next writing project is to be "Crying Out to God, in the Manner of the Lord's Prayer."

A couple of years ago I published an article with Ezine "How to cry out to God" and the phrase "crying out to God" through search engines has received more than 1,400 hits on the article.

75 October 24, 2012 Wednesday

I visited with the senior warden of Trinity Church for sorting out what administrative decisions are required to be made by November 15th for EfM first year to start in January. She was very helpful.

These are the executive decisions I've made:

1. Admit to the group only first year students because it would be too demanding for me to prepare for more than one year at a time
2. Have Diane sign papers.
3. Send in all the enrollment papers together.
4. I am to make an announcement in church inviting those interested in the program to meet with me at coffee.
5. Senior Warden assisted me in drawing up a list of individuals to invite to the program.

I'm surprised how easily I moved into the executive role – it's a very new place for me to be. I've failed in this role a number of times, new question to ask, "What executive decisions do I find necessary?"

76 November 11, 2012 Saturday

Instead of journaling, I've been praying in my prayer journals using what I learned in the bishop's retreat led by Sybil MacBeth.

The 2012 general election was on November 6th. The Presidential Election cycle ends an important cycle in David's and my life. On Monday and Tuesday I was remembering David's telling me to remarry when he was gone, and then *I took my wedding band off Tuesday night. Wednesday morning I started wearing my 50th anniversary ring on my right hand.*

Not knowing that eventually it would become our anniversary ring, I had purchased it in the gift shop at Mt. Rushmore. The ring is made from Black Hills gold, and has four grape leaves intertwined, two yellow and two pink, symbolic of love intertwined, of religious faith and also the sacredness of marriage. David and I were at Mt. Rushmore a few years before we moved to Idaho. I was using an electric scooter and taking the Parkinson's meds and we were on our way to visit our Pocatello family. Shortly after our frightening double diagnoses in 2010, I had a diamond placed at the middle juncture of two of the grape leaves.

The following year in May we had an anniversary celebration at the care facility. It was then that I decided that the ring would be for our 50th anniversary. Our 50th anniversary would be in December of that year but we observed it during Memorial Day Weekend. Philip and his older daughter Heather came. Paula and her family were there. We reserved the table in the alcove of the dining room and we had a Thanksgiving feast with turkey and all the rest. David was wheeled from the memory care unit. David enjoyed us all being there and having thanksgiving and our anniversary. We even had a 50th anniversary cake. He smiled and laughed and managed to talk a little.

77 November 16, 2012 Friday

So what would happen if I stopped trying to write E-books? I find so much resistance within myself. What would happen if I re-invented my life? What would it look like? I'm depressed. I slip my wedding ring back on my finger.

78 November 17, 2012 Saturday

This morning I prayed on my depression. Insights came and at 4 pm I turned on Garrison Keillor. I haven't listened to him in ages. In his monologue about Lake Woebegone he talked about the Lutheran minister's homily of "The Widow's Half Penny." She gave out of her poverty. "If you are depressed, give a party. If you feel insecure, give someone security."

In prayer I diagramed a word cluster with "give from your poverty" at the center. From this center rays fanned out:

- Feel like an outsider in a social situation? Focus on one person and ask questions about her/his life.
- Depressed? Ask someone to do something with you.
- Insecure? Give security to someone through acts of mercy.
- Shy? Give hope to someone.
- Regrets? Forgive yourself as God has forgiven you.
- Procrastinator? Make plans with someone.
- Alone or Lonely? Make friends, nurture existing friendships.
- Want to hide? Walk out in the open, connect with someone.
- Hard to do anything? Do things in blocks of 30 minutes or less.

The homily pointed out that the widow gave everything she had. Jesus pointed her out to the disciples in contrast to the other people who gave from their abundance.

There is an application to my writing also. God blesses and multiplies what I give to his use.

79 November 24, 2012 Saturday

Thanksgiving Day was fine due to my involvement with Paula and Tad's large gathering of friends and Paula's students.

I'm thinking forward to the annual Messiah Sing at Stevens Auditorium. The last time I went was in 2010. I took David and we sat in the tenor section. He wouldn't allow me to help him. Instead he turned to the young man next to him who guided David to the pages in the score.

I will ask Trent and Chris from church to accompany me.

Yesterday I was busy with creating my author page on Goodreads and then in the afternoon I played Scrabble with a new acquaintance.

Today I'm feeling the loss of David. The grief has been running underground in the midst of busyness. I want to join him so badly. The thought has occurred to me several times to purchase a hand gun, go someplace and shoot either my heart or at my head in the temple. I would leave a note so my body could be found. Will I do it? NO!

I turn to the journal entries for the last few days of David's life and am comforted. I feel connected to him.

The widow's job is to stay alive.

80 December 17, 2012 Monday

David,

I feel free to talk to you now. Last night I chose not to go to the Messiah even though I was going with Trent and Chris. A big storm was supposedly coming through to dump 6 inches of snow in Pocatello, so I gave my regrets and stayed home.

CNN was broadcasting from Newtown, Connecticut regarding the massacre of twenty 6 and 7 year olds in their school. There was a community wide service held in the high school auditorium arranged by the religious leaders – Jewish, Muslim, Ba Hai, Catholic, and Protestant faiths. Our dear President Obama spoke.

Our hearts are broken.

What is it like when the souls of these innocent little ones come to Heaven? Is there joyful welcoming? Sadness on their loss of life?

David, watch over me and pray for me. I love you and I long to be re-united with you.

Judy

81 December 25, 2012 Tuesday – Christmas Day

David,

I feel your loss more on Christmas, more than a year ago. I feel empty, sad, alone. I don't want to go on, but I will for your sake. Each day is an active choice to be alive, some days more than others. The waves of grief are crashing over me – the Christmas season is the most difficult.

Judy

Hope, love, joy and peace are the themes of this season.

- Hope: I do have hope that all who mourn this season will be comforted.
- Love: *Lord, let me feel your love while I miss the hugs of my dear one.*
- Joy: I hear and see joy around me, but I'm not experiencing joy. I trust that once again joy will be with me.
- Peace: I feel peace when I resolve regrets, when I experience forgiveness, and when I help others.

I was surprised by the question that came to me this morning *"Do you want to be happy?"*

I was further surprised by my answer *"No."*

What is this question and answer about? Is there a way to couple "happy" and "grief" as with "good" and "grief"?

Lord, help me to resolve my grief and to fully accept the loss of my husband. Help me to experience joy and happiness once again.

What will be helpful?

- Write and publish
- Blog and Facebook
- Log each day's blessings, gratitude, joy, and happiness
- Be sociable
- Journal
- Bible meditation and prayer

Catch the fleeting moments of feeling comforted, blessed, a sense of joy, happiness and being grateful. Catch the moments of being aware of God's Presence.

82   December 26, 2012 Wednesday

David,

I feel guilty that I wasn't the one to die first. Never thought I would experience Survivor's Guilt, but here it is. I feel this way because you were such a good person and I am terribly flawed. But dying is not about being good or flawed, nor calling us home. Death comes by natural means or by human action. I believe God welcomes us home with peace and joy.

I love you.

Today's log:

I'm thankful for a good day, the heaviness has lifted. I enjoy Brenda's company and conversation as cleans my apartment. I feel blessed by her. I'm thrilled with the progress I'm making on "Abuse Survivors: Self-Guided Retreat." I'm revising the published book as I go. I was social by bringing a tray of fruit for tea time at Cardona Senior Apartments. I've experienced happiness today.

83 December 27, 2012 Thursday

David,

I'm feeling pretty good today. I had coffee with artist George Wise. He kindly read my manuscript "Crying Out to God." He says for believers, the prayers open doors. David, your insistence for me to keep writing keeps me going.

I love you.

Today's log:

I'm thankful for a good day and being able to be sociable with George Wise, Ralph and Grant at coffee this morning in Old Town. I'm grateful that I could be sociable at Cardona Senior Apartments. I'm very thankful for Richard Lemon's expertise in Physical Therapy. My neck is doing well, lower back has improved, but still iffy and will continue to be compromised from severe spinal stenosis also termed spinal spondylosis. I've had to give up my goals of walking 4 miles, bicycling and lifting 50 lbs. I'm not able to climb steps because of severe pain in my right knee.

84   January 6, 2013 Sunday - Epiphany

Two years ago, David and I walked into Trinity Church for the first time. Today I could enter the liturgy with fresh sensitivities, listen to the story of The Three Kings with new understanding, and the homily touched me at so many levels.

David dear, the story of the birth of Jesus in a manger, meager simple stable and yet a guiding star the magi who were not Jewish were led to the new born baby. They who were outsiders brought the gifts, the symbols of Christ's call to the world to be humble, nonviolent, embracing all of humanity, a teacher by living the spiritual path of the unification of all peoples.

David you heard the story and the glorious Epiphany music and you came home to your beginning as a Christian growing up in the Roman Catholic Church. You loved being at Trinity Church that day, in participating, singing and receiving Communion. You were welcomed home.

Judy

85 January 11, 2013 Friday

Lots of snow yesterday and today, all schools closed including ISU. Temps tonight will be minus zero degrees.

Philip and Paula are in Pittsburgh this weekend to be with Grandma Brutz, David's mother. Kate, age 97, had a stroke on New Year's Day. Prognosis is actually good since she regained speech and asked to be taken off her feeding tube.

86 January 14, 2013 Monday

"Now is the day of salvation" (2 Corinthians 6:2)

The scripture listed for today's entry in Upper Room and the focus is for people who are thinking about suicide. My prayer focus became **"Save me from self-destruction."**

87   January 16, 2012 Wednesday

Yesterday I added a new page, "Praying" to my website.

Today I had a long conversation with a friend who is moving away. The conversation became a reality check for me when my friend spoke about experiencing me as a person who pushes hard in everything I do. It is true. The phrase *"I need to stop pushing" keeps showing up in my journal. My body is letting me know that I must stop pushing. The damage from spondylosis in my spine cannot be undone. It is worse. I'm older and I'm tired.*

What does this mean practically? Stop signing up for adult education and Workforce classes. It is okay for me to stay home several days in a row and work on my writing projects and take naps.

88   January 26, 2013 Saturday

The 24th was David's birthday and I've observed the day by making oatmeal for breakfast like he did every morning for decades, with cinnamon, raisins and walnuts; except I substituted craisins for raisins. This might be a good thing to do when I'm hit with a wave of grief – good to do on Christmas and our anniversary too.

89 February 19, 2013 Tuesday

Today was my third session of acupuncture with Ethan, a talented acupuncturist. I was amazed how I could work with the chi flow using my energy practice from Healing Touch and Reiki. It has taken three sessions for the energy to flow freely.

Between taking meds for depression and anxiety and having acupuncture, I'm feeling free in mind and spirit. I feel happy. I'm singing. I'm laughing and I'm initiating conversations.

90 March 2, 2013 Saturday

Husband dear, I miss you. I love you. I want to be with you. Thank you for accepting me. We have fond memories.

91   March 9, 2013 Saturday

I'm exhausted tonight. It has been a busy week with appointments, working on my "Crying Out to God" manuscript and in communicating with Create Space.

I've learned how to create a cover using a Create Space template. The learning curve has been sharp. I'm thrilled to have accomplished creating this book. Next week I will order 50 copies.

The fun highlight this week was going with Paula and her husband Tad to see "The Susical Musical" at Pocatello High, Julia was one of the dancers. The production was excellent and the dancing and singing were superb. As always, Julia danced with enthusiasm. I laughed a lot.

Next week will be filled with appointments including having work done on the Prius and having my taxes done by an AARP volunteer at Marshall Public Library.

This week I returned the papers from Council Gardens indicating that I am withdrawing my name from the waiting list.

I've decided to stay in Pocatello because of the many friends and networks I have, the excellent housing at Cardona, the mountains, the wilderness and especially because of Trinity Episcopal Church. David wants me to stay here and go to this church. And now I have the additional reason which

Paula points out, the cost of living in Pocatello is much lower than in Cleveland, Ohio. I am not able to afford living in Cleveland.

Regarding another decision I've made this week, David influences my thinking in regard whether to attend the Annual Gathering of Friends General Conference which will be in Greenly, Colorado this summer. He would tell me that I should go while I am still able and its location is close enough to drive.

92 March 12, 2013 Tuesday

Draggy and tired today, I'm doing too much. It is difficult to slow down since I've been experiencing more energy lately but I am 72 years old.

I found out that the cost of living in Cleveland is 41% higher than in Pocatello. This is the bottom line about any possibility to relocate. The likelihood of increasing my income that amount is nil.

Yesterday I approved the review file for "Crying Out to God." I purchased copies and both it and my first book will be available at Trinity on Deanery Day. The shipment will arrive on March 15th.

Today I went online and applied for an Idaho Sales Permit. The sales tax in Idaho is 6%.

In regard to my spinal stenosis (spondylosis) I asked Ethan if the acupuncture will help stabilize my condition. He says it is highly possible but it will take a while for the brain to get the message of what it is suppose to do and that is why it is important to stay on top of it through consistent treatments. Dr. Joseph my orthopedist agrees with Ethan.

93   March 13, 2013 Wednesday

The College of Cardinals today chose the next pope who is taking the name of Francis (of Assisi). I'm thrilled.

David dear, I know you would be pleased because he is humble person who like Pope John XXIII embraces the poor and all of humanity. Taking the name of Francis speaks volumes.

Well, my dear, goodnight and my blessings. I love you and long to be with you in Heaven.

94 March 26, 2013 Tuesday

I'm pleased that acupuncture treatments are helping to improve my walking. Ethan, my acupuncturist, is having me come in once a week. When I saw orthopedist Dr. Joseph last week he was ready to release me. He said my knees would continue to improve during April from the shots. Already today I am able to go up and down stairs at Cardona without pain, not even soreness. The exercise I do at PT is greatly strengthening all the muscles in my legs and buttocks. That makes a difference in doing stairs.

This evening I phoned Philip to inform him that I wouldn't be relocating to Cleveland Heights due to the cost of living. He became loud and kept repeating himself challenging what the cost of living was based on. His thinking is that since Council Gardens includes subsidized housing the difference in cost of living wouldn't affect me.

I left the conversation realizing that the middle of my chest was hurting. It took me a while to admit that I was having a panic attach. I took a half tablet of anti-anxiety meds and soon the physical feeling left as well as the mental and emotional affect.

In the midst of the attack I felt very guilty as though I was rejecting my son. The truth is I don't want to leave Pocatello. Why couldn't I say that instead of pinning my decision based on the cost of living? I have made a life here. I have friends and acquaintances. I'm in the Rocky Mountains and I don't want to leave them. I'm in a church I love in which my gifts are recognized and used.

95 April 7, 2013 Sunday

I feel at home in Trinity. I feel David's presence. I want to stay in Pocatello because of Trinity. I want to stay in Pocatello because David and I came here together, because we love one another, and because I recall things he said.

"Don't even question whether to go to church, just do it."

When we were much younger he read the Philip's translation of the New Testament. When the Roman Catholic Church allowed lay readers, David was one of the first to read the lessons at St Augustine where we lived on the Near West Side of Cleveland.

David took to heart from early childhood to love Jesus and follow him. He didn't mouth the teachings of Christ, he lived them. As a single man he went on retreats. He had a devotion to Mary and prayed the rosary privately. He stopped doing these practices after we left the church.

I feel I failed David miserably in our marriage. However, in the last few months of his life we came together holding one another. We experienced forgiveness and our love blossomed into full maturity.

Thank you God, for reconciliation through Jesus the Mediator and for grace through the Holy Spirit.

96 May 2, 2013 Thursday

I'm drawn into too many directions – forever true. How to order my life?

Lord, help me to order my life.

- Caring for myself

  4 hours of PT per week

  Acupuncture once a week

  Physical care and nutrition
- Spiritual and emotional care

  Church every Sunday

  Prayer
- Writing – I must write everyday for at least an hour

I have three ministries:

1. Writing – takes priority over the other ministries
2. Mentoring – beginning in September, mentoring the first year of Education for Ministry (EfM)
3. Pastoral care through Trinity

And still I reiterate to myself that writing must come first. I let distractions get in the way such as Facebook. I love to post photos of nature, birds, and animals because my spirits are lifted by viewing creation. Also it lifts my spirits to post a blessing each evening. Another distraction is watching evening TV programs. At least I examine my conscience on whether this is an evening for TV instead of something else.

Each week everything must be built around PT, acupuncture, and writing.

97   June 1, 2013 Saturday

I began this volume of my journal August 26, 2011 just a few days before David died. I am now at the end of the volume and not wanting to run out of space to write nor to move on. Am I ready to move on?

Three years ago David was diagnosed with Glioblastoma Multiforme. This anniversary of his diagnosis brings with it a smashing wave of grief.

98   July 7, 2013 Sunday – Laramie, Wyoming

I'm returning from the 2013 Gathering of Friends General Conference in Greely, Colorado. The scenery as I drive is spectacular – the geology in particular. As I drive I'm thinking of David, he would be commenting on the geology and we would be stopping at every point of interest. I'm enjoying my thoughts of David.

For me to be driving this long trip is an achievement – it is the first road trip I've driven alone since David died and I can do it!

At the Gathering I was fortunate to be able to secure a spot in John Calvi's workshop. I learned in John's workshop "Abandon All Weariness" to give myself facial and foot massages, and reminded to do Healing Touch on myself daily. Why do I abandon these practices? John reinforced the importance of paying attention to what our bodies are telling us which affirms my need for PT and acupuncture. John suggests that I cry for two hours a week. Why am I reluctant to cry? Why will I not take his advice and read or view movies which bring tears? I can say this – everyone grieves in their own way and in their own time, everyone is unique and yet grief is universal.

In regard to participating in the Gathering of FGC, I conclude that it is important for me to go to the annual Gathering as long as the travel is feasible. At the Gathering I reconnect in person with Friends (Quakers) I know who come from all over the country and Canada. So many of whom I have known for decades.

I would like to lead a workshop for the 2014 Gathering and to that end I will put in a proposal due at the end of September.

99 July 14, 2013 Sunday

Today I was received into the Episcopal Church by Bishop Brian Thom, Bishop of the Diocese of Idaho, at Trinity Church in Pocatello. I'm thrilled. I've come to rest in the Episcopal Church and to continue my affiliation with the Religious Society of Friends. I choose dual affiliation.

100   August 15, 2013 Thursday

On this date in 1962, I was baptized as an adult in the Roman Catholic Church in Boston. I was baptized on the Feast Day of Mary's Assumption into Heaven. I was given the baptismal name of Judith Maria. I was pregnant and a little more than two weeks later Philip was born at "Boston Lying in Hospital" now named "Brigham Women and Children's Hospital."

I was baptized at St. Joseph's next to Massachusetts General Hospital - the church was later torn down to make way for the hospital's expansion. The following spring, I was confirmed in the faith by Cardinal Cushing in the Cathedral.

David was pleased with my conversion and baptism. Every Sunday and Feast Days we went to Mass together and shared the Missal which had Latin on one page and English on the facing one. We prayed the Rosary side-by-side in church. We were observant Catholics. That changed when we left the Church during the Viet Nam War and found Friends (Quakers). We were with Friends until we walked into Trinity Episcopal Church when David was declining from brain cancer.

None of us know where our spiritual journey will take us, which twists and turns might occur. I do know that my journey deepens my faith and closeness to God and that living Love is my lifelong path.

To My Dearest Love

September 5, 2013 Thursday

My Dearest Love,

Today is the second anniversary of your dying. I began the day by making Oatmeal with raisins, walnuts, and cinnamon. I soaked the raisin briefly not overnight the way you were accustomed to doing nor did I search for their stems to pick off. The Oatmeal tasted so good and brought back memories of your making Oatmeal each morning, for how many decades?

There came a point, possibly when we lived in Des Moines that you started buying 50 lb bags of old fashion steel cut oats. You stored the bag in the basement in a large metal garbage can with a tight fitting lid. You continued this practice when we moved to Pocatello, but then stopped, and I'm not sure when or why.

I seemed to be oblivious to most everything when I was being treated for Parkinson's. The medications produced a mental fog as well as personality changes. Then later when I was being treated for Hepatitis C instead of PD, I was in a medication induced fog as well.

How patient and caring you were. Sometime during that period you began to have mental changes – you became more eccentric, more adamant that everything had to be done in an exact way; drove me nuts. How did we ever pull through? But we did make the transition through the Holy One's Love and care for us. We were blessed in our relationship, our marriage of fifty years.

Today Sally and her grown kids, Michelle and John, had me over for lunch so that I would be with someone on your anniversary. We played Scrabble and I thoroughly enjoyed myself.

This evening I changed my profile and cover photos on Facebook from you and me sitting together on the Alaskan train to my author photo for the profile picture and from the Alaskan Glacier to the photo of Philip and his family with me at Yellowstone for the cover photo. I feel so good about these changes that perhaps I'm ready to move on - better to say that transition continues.

Other markers that the transition continues is my sustained urge to downsize, to recycle what I no longer need or use – everything from books, clothes, documents to stored stuff.

I love you David.

***

The first time I saw David was at St. John's College in Annapolis, Maryland in September of 1959. It was the first day of the school year and the College welcomed the students by having a sit-down dinner replete with white linen

184

table cloths and napkins, and student waiters dressed in white jackets and black bowties. (Yes, all the waiters were guys.) We sat at round tables seating eight. I was a first year student, and was taking everything in.

The face of a waiter, a few tables away, caught my attention. There was a light and gentleness that radiated from him. I studied his face and turned to the woman next to me.

"There is a good person."

Later, I learned that "he" was David Brutz, and that when he waited tables he meditated on Thomas A Kempis' *"The Imitation of Christ."*

Whenever I saw him walking in my direction, I would deviate from the walkway. It took several months before I actually had a conversation with him. We talked about classical music; he was the sound guy for the College. One day, he was coming in from the outside when I was coming down a flight of stairs. I sat down on a step while David crouched on the floor. Oh, my, was he ever handsome, and yet, I was not ready for a relationship.

On Saturday nights there were two parties on campus, one was in the boat house and included loud music and booze. I neither drank nor cared for loud music. The other party was the "waltz party" which took place in the Great Hall - no booze, and only beautiful Viennese waltzes. The students who went to the Great Hall tended to be quiet and polite. I occasionally went there.

During the second semester, I danced with David, yet, I continued to feel shy. It's a wonder we ever got together. We became good friends, and it was the end of the second summer that we began to realize the significance of our relationship. David proposed in the fall and we drove to Walden Pond and married each other, and then petitioned Rome to allow us to marry during Advent. We were married on December 9, 1961 in Boston, Massachusetts.

I had to become willing to having a relationship with David because I was a Quaker pacifist and he was a Catholic who had served four years in the army, albeit peacetime. As a Friend (Quaker) I believed that there was no need for an intermediator between myself and God. It was okay for David to be Catholic, but when the priest, in interviewing us, told David that he was to pray and work for my conversion, and David agreed- that was another matter.

Afterwards, we went to my apartment.

"David, how could you have agreed to work and pray for my conversion?" I was clearly distraught. "I can't accept this."

With teary eyes, my dear David got up to leave. I was crying. What was I doing?

"No, David, don't leave. Please, don't leave."

Dear Lord,

Even though we walk through the shadow of death
You are with us.

Hold us close and comfort our aching hearts
With your Love guide us through our grief.

Fill us with hope that
Mourning will give way to joy.

Acknowledgments

I appreciate the caring and prayers from my loved ones and friends. I'm grateful to the health care professionals who tended to both my husband and me during our respective illnesses. Thanks to the people of Trinity Episcopal Church in Pocatello for embracing us. I'm grateful to our dear friend, Dr. Roger Boe, for your caring encouragement during the writing process, and to author Pam Mosbrucker for her mentoring.

About the Author

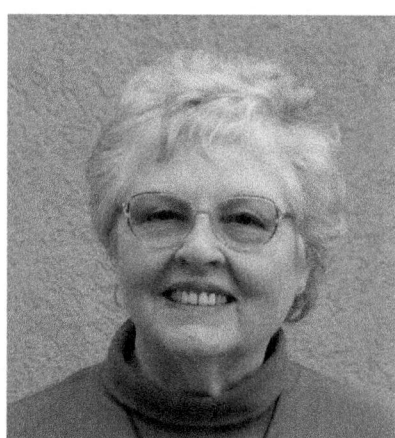

Photo by artist George White

Judy Brutz, PhD, AAMFT is a graduate of Iowa State University in Ames, Iowa. Her career spans marriage and family therapy, education, pastoral counseling, hospice chaplaincy, spiritual direction and retreat leadership. In retirement, her ministry is in giving encouragement through her writing, pastoral care, teaching, speaking, retreat leadership, and mentoring in the Education for Ministry (EfM) program.

Author's Website and Blog: www.judybrutz.com
Author's Facebook Page:
www.facebook.com/Judy.Brutz.Author

If you are interested in engaging Judy Brutz for a speaking event or retreat leadership, please contact her through her website or Author Page at Facebook.

Pine River Press, Pocatello, Idaho
Publishes the works of Judy Brutz

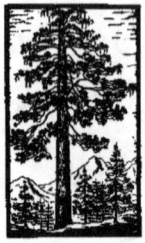

www.pineriverpress.com

www.ingramcontent.com/pod-product-compliance
Lightning Source LLC
Chambersburg PA
CBHW070902290526
45795CB00001B/209